Step by Step®
Urticaria & Angioedema Management

Step by Step®
Urticaria & Angioedema Management

Second Edition

Sanjay Ghosh MD
Former Professor and Head
Department of Dermatology
MGM Medical College and LSK Hospital
Kishanganj, Bihar
Former Medical Director (Honorary)
Institute of Allergic and Immunologic Skin Diseases
Kolkata, West Bengal, India

Saurav Kundu MD
Professor
Department of Dermatology
MGM Medical College and LSK Hospital
Kishanganj, Bihar, India

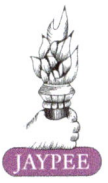

JAYPEE
JAYPEE BROTHERS MEDICAL PUBLISHERS
The Health Sciences Publisher
New Delhi | London

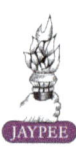

Jaypee Brothers Medical Publishers (P) Ltd

Headquarters
EMCA House
23/23-B, Ansari Road, Daryaganj
New Delhi 110 002, India
Landline: +91-11-23272143
+91-11-23272703, +91-11-23282021
+91-11-23245672
E-mail: jaypee@jaypeebrothers.com

Corporate Office
Jaypee Brothers Medical Publishers (P) Ltd.
4838/24, Ansari Road, Daryaganj
New Delhi 110 002, India
Phone: +91-11-43574357
Fax: +91-11-43574314
E-mail: jaypee@jaypeebrothers.com

Overseas Office
JP Medical Ltd.
83, Victoria Street, London
SW1H 0HW (UK)
Phone: +44-20 3170 8910
E-mail: info@jpmedpub.com

EU GPSR Authorised Representative
Logos Europe, 9 rue Nicolas Poussin
17000, La Rochelle, France
Phone: +33 (0) 6 67 93 73 78
E-mail: Contact@logoseurope.eu

Website: www.jaypeebrothers.com
Website: www.jaypeedigital.com

© 2024, Jaypee Brothers Medical Publishers

The views and opinions expressed in this book are solely those of the original contributor(s)/author(s) and do not necessarily represent those of editor(s) or publisher of the book.

All rights reserved. No part of this publication may be reproduced, stored or transmitted in any form or by any means, electronic, mechanical, photocopying, recording or otherwise, without the prior permission in writing of the publishers.

All brand names and product names used in this book are trade names, service marks, trademarks or registered trademarks of their respective owners. The publisher is not associated with any product or vendor mentioned in this book.

Medical knowledge and practice change constantly. This book is designed to provide accurate, authoritative information about the subject matter in question. However, readers are advised to check the most current information available on procedures included and check information from the manufacturer of each product to be administered, to verify the recommended dose, formula, method and duration of administration, adverse effects and contraindications. It is the responsibility of the practitioner to take all appropriate safety precautions. Neither the publisher nor the author(s)/editor(s) assume any liability for any injury and/or damage to persons or property arising from or related to use of material in this book.

This book is sold on the understanding that the publisher is not engaged in providing professional medical services. If such advice or services are required, the services of a competent medical professional should be sought.

Every effort has been made where necessary to contact holders of copyright to obtain permission to reproduce copyright material. If any have been inadvertently overlooked, the publisher will be pleased to make the necessary arrangements at the first opportunity.

Inquiries for bulk sales may be solicited at: jaypee@jaypeebrothers.com

Step by Step® Urticaria & Angioedema Management / Sanjay Ghosh, Saurav Kundu

First Edition: 2016

Second Edition: 2024

ISBN: 978-93-5696-982-7

Dedicated to
All our urticaria patients

Preface to the Second Edition

The first edition of this book got amazing response from dermatologists, both students and practitioners, and we received repeated requests from readers of different sectors to update the book. That is why we have been prompted to bring out this new edition.

Urticaria is a subject where new research findings are being obtained almost each and every day and newer modalities and approaches are coming very frequently for the management of the disease. Hence, a book on this subject needs regular editing. Due to our professional hectic schedules and innumerable personal commitments, we were not able to bring the newer version earlier for which we feel extremely sorry and request our dear readers to excuse us.

For working out this new edition, we are thankful to the whole team of Jaypee Brothers Medical Publishers for supporting wholeheartedly.

Last but not least, we will be grateful to our readers if they love the book and get benefited from its content. We will be obliged to get suggestions from our readers for improvisation of future editions.

Sanjay Ghosh
Saurav Kundu

Preface to the First Edition

Urticaria has been one of the most common skin ailments of human beings and increasing in galloping rates in recent decades. Therapeutic approach in urticaria remains always difficult and challenging in spite of better understanding of its pathogenesis and clinical spectrum in present time. Typifying the urticaria would be the cornerstone in the proper management of urticaria as different variety may need more specific medication and prevention. Therapy in urticaria advances everyday with newer drugs and regimens or guidelines but controversies always prevail.

In this backdrop the entity, urticaria demands a concise book on its own with updated information for ready reference of the busy dermatology practitioners who may not get adequate time always to touch the subject in details. That was the main object of composing this book which does not necessarily claim to cover the subject exhaustively. If the readers find the book useful for their purpose we would feel our efforts not to go in vain.

We acknowledge and express our sincere regards to Shri Jitendar P Vij (Group Chairman), Mr Ankit Vij (Managing Director), Mr Tarun Duneja (Director–Publishing) and all the team members of M/S Jaypee Brothers Medical Publishers (P) Ltd, New Delhi, India for the eagerness to continue this book, regular support and cooperation in every step of publishing this book.

Sanjay Ghosh
Saurav Kundu

Contents

1. **Urticaria**   1
   Definition *1*
   History *5*
   Epidemiology *6*
   Etiopathogenesis *6*
   Classification *9*
   Quality of Life *11*
   Clinical Features *11*
   Symptomatic Dermographism *18*
   Differential Diagnosis *37*
   Annexure *48*

2. **Angioedema**   51
   Definition *51*
   Etiopathological Classification *52*
   Pathophysiology *52*
   Clinical Features *57*
   Investigations *58*
   Angioedema Activity Score *59*

3. **Urticarial Syndromes**   60
   Familial *61*
   Familial Urticarial Syndromes *61*
   Nonfamilial Autoinflammatory Diseases *63*

4. **Management**   65
   Acute Urticaria *65*
   Chronic Urticaria *66*
   Cyclosporine *79*
   Topical Corticosteroids *80*
   Angioedema *83*

Bibliography   85
Index   89

CHAPTER 1

Urticaria

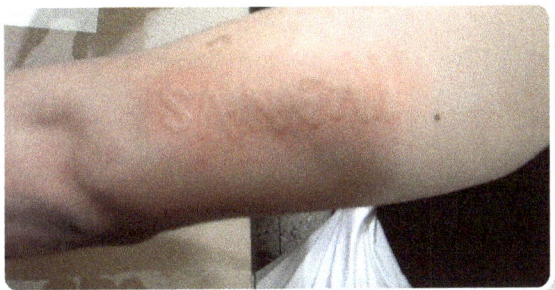

Definition

- Urticaria is characterized by the rapid appearance of wheals with or without *angioedema*.

Wheal comprises of
- A central edematous swelling of variable size, almost invariably surrounded by a reflex erythema
- Associated itching or sometimes burning sensation
- A fleeting nature with the skin returning to its normal appearance usually within 1–24 hours
- Upper or mid-dermal swelling **(Figs. 1.1 and 1.2)**

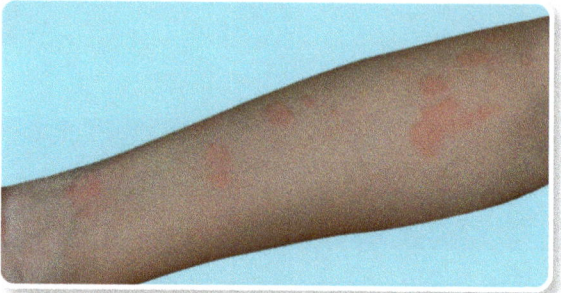

Fig. 1.1: Typical wheals.

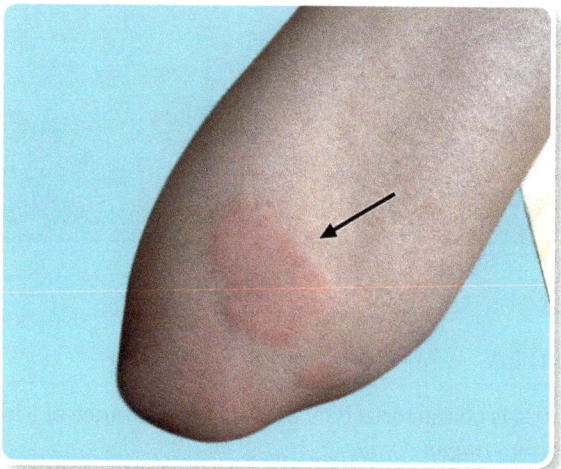

Fig. 1.2: A typical wheal on elbow.

Angioedema is characterized by
- Sudden marked swelling of the lower dermis and subcutis
- Sometimes pain rather than itching
- Frequent involvement of the mucous membrane
- Resolution that is slower than for wheals, which can take up to 72 hours **(Figs. 1.3 to 1.7)**

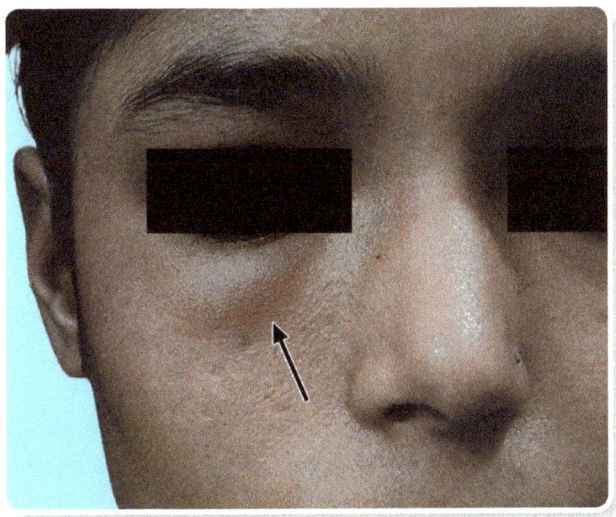

Fig. 1.3: A typical angioedema on face.

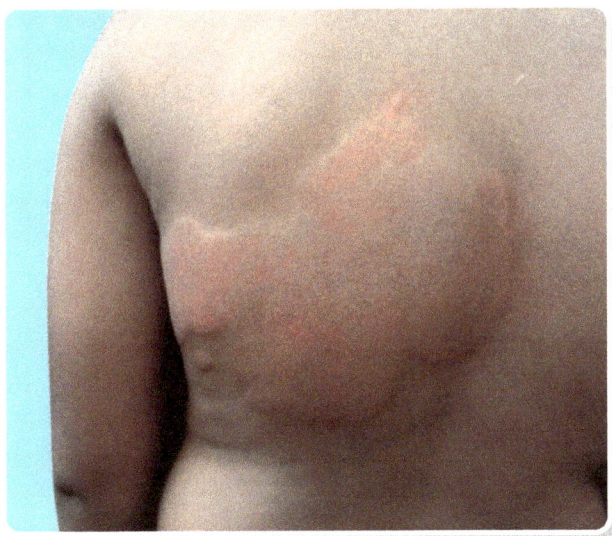

Fig. 1.4: A typical angioedema on back.

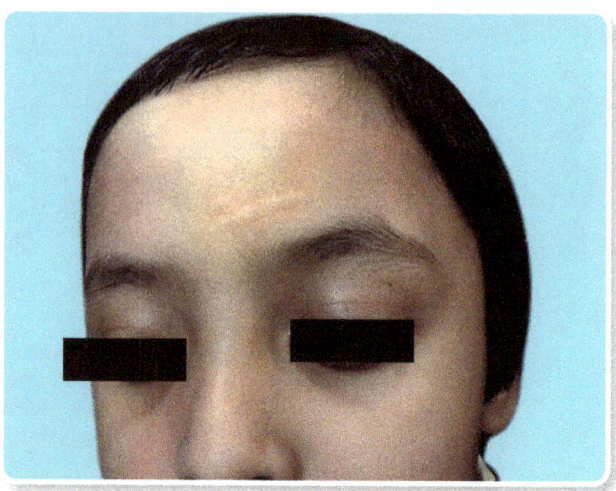

Fig. 1.5: Urticaria and angioedema in a child.

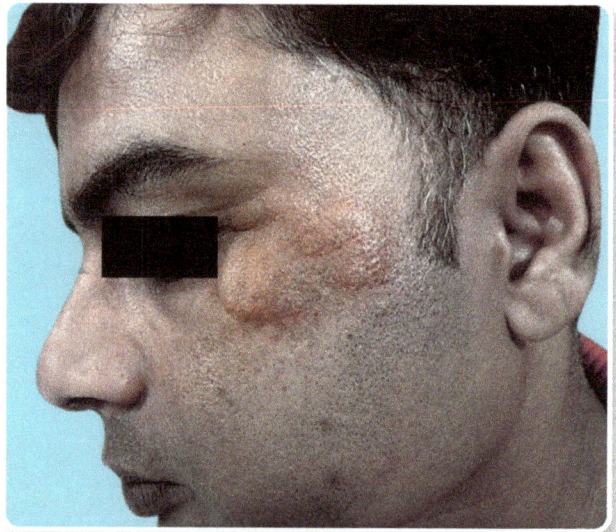

Fig. 1.6: Angioedema on left side of face.

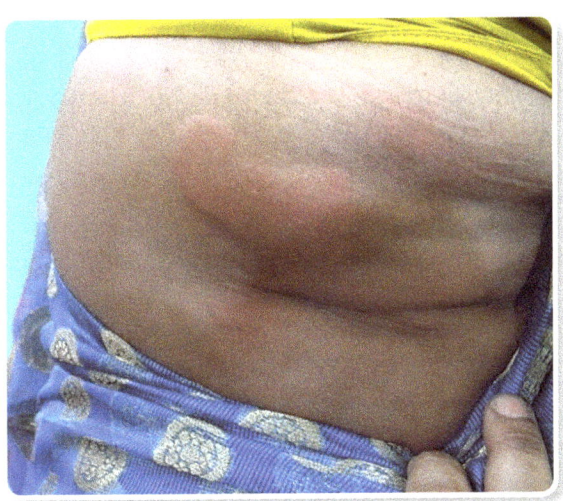

Fig. 1.7: Angioedema on side of chest.

Comparison between *wheals* and *angioedema*:

Wheals	Angioedema
Superficial dermis	Deep dermis/subcutis/mucosa
Last for several hours	Last for several days
Hand and feet	Head region, hand, and feet

History

- Clinical descriptions of urticaria have been found in the writings of Hippocrates in the 4th century BC to Heberden and Willan at the end of the 18th century AD.
- The pathophysiological era is dawned by the discovery of mast cell (mastzellen) by Paul Erlich in 1877.
- Mast cell as a source of histamine was identified by Riley and West.
- Histamine was discovered by Dale in 1906 from extracts of ergot and described all important actions of histamine.
- Lewis first outlined the potency of histamine as a mediator of wealing in human skin.
- The characterization of reaginic immunoglobulin E (IgE) by Ishizaka enabled the understanding of autoallergic urticaria but the pathogenesis of chronic idiopathic urticaria remained obscure.

- The autologous serum skin test by Grattan in 1986 first demonstrated that the cause of chronic urticaria was endogenous. However, the factors such as dysregulation of intracellular signal transducer in mast cell and basophils are also important.

Epidemiology

- Around 15-20% of people have urticaria at least once during their lifetime.
- There is no age bar for urticaria or angioedema although urticaria is mostly seen after adolescence.
- The highest incidence of urticaria is seen in young adults.
- Exact epidemiology of chronic urticaria in India is not known. Worldwide, it occurs in 0.1-3% of the population.
- Women are twice commonly affected compared to men.

Etiopathogenesis

- Urticaria is a disease with varied clinical presentations and etiologies.
- The clinical patterns and the triggers guide the physician to investigate and manage the individual appropriately.
- Most types of urticaria are due to promiscuous activation of mast cells, although basophils are also involved.
- Histologically, wheals are characterized by edema of upper and mid-dermis with dilatation of postcapillary venules whereas in angioedema mainly lower dermis and subcutis is affected. There is a mixed cellular infiltrate of both acute and chronic inflammatory cells. Different cells and the mediator pathways, which play a pivotal role in urticaria, have been discussed below.
- The inflammatory profiles of the skin of chronic spontaneous urticaria (CSU) patients (wheals and nonlesional sites) and healthy controls are different. Cells like mast cells, eosinophils, and basophils interact, release vasoactive mediators, and sensitize the skin, which predisposes the patients to develop symptoms. In these inflammatory cascades, many cytokines and chemokines are involved who may trigger their corresponding intracellular signaling. From these understanding, development of therapies such as omalizumab, dupilumab, and Bruton's tyrosine kinase (BTK) inhibitors was possible.

- CSU cases are mostly due to immunologic mechanisms of mast cell (MC) activation. Two such mechanisms may contribute to the pathogenesis of CSU; however, sometimes they may overlap. The extracellular α-subunit of the high-affinity IgE receptor (FcεRI), the predominant part of the receptor that is exposed at the surface of MCs and basophils are involved in both the mechanisms. FcεRI may also be important factor in the pathogenesis of chronic inducible urticaria, but the triggering factors are different.
- A type I autoimmune response is often characterized as an autoallergic response. The key to autoallergy is the presence of an autoantigen in the skin that can form a complex with IgE and activate MCs. A type IIb autoimmune response is one in which IgG and possibly IgM antibodies to FcεRI or IgE cross-link FcεRI or FcεRI-bound IgE, respectively.

> *On the basis of etiopathogenesis, urticaria can be*
> - Histaminergic, i.e., mediated by histamine
> - Nonhistaminergic, i.e., mediated by bradykinin

Histaminergic

- Mast cell is the key effector cell of acute and chronic urticaria. Studies using conventional histochemical stains show mast cell predominance in urticarial lesions.
- Among the mediators released during mast cells degranulation histamine and leukotrienes, LTC4, D4, and E4 appear to be most important.
- Roles of heparin and tryptase remain unclear.
- Histamine is mainly responsible for the wheals and itch whereas flare is mediated by substance P.
- LTC4, D4, and E4 play an important role in nonselective nonsteroidal antiinflammatory drugs (NSAIDs) induced urticaria which result in diversion of arachidonic acid metabolism from PGE2 to leukotrienes. The reduced PGE2 level has a permissive effect on immunological mast cell degranulation. That is not seen with selective cyclooxygenase-2 (COX-2) inhibitors **(Fig. 1.8)**.
- Other cells which play an important role in the late phase of urticaria has been shown in **Table 1.1**.

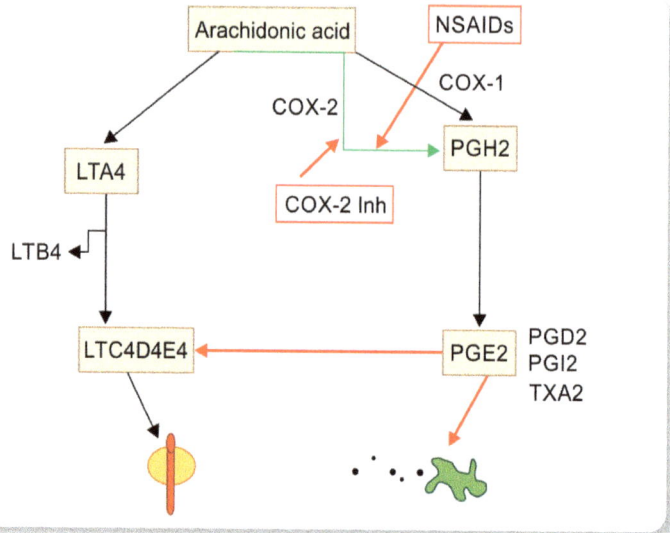

Fig. 1.8: Inhibition of cyclooxygenase (COX) pathway. NSAIDs blocks COX pathway leading to diversion of arachidonic acid metabolism from prostaglandins to leukotrienes. PGE2 normally inhibits immunological mast cell degranulation and leukotriene production. Low PGE2 formation by NSAIDs encourages immunological mast cell degranulations. Selective COX-2 inhibitor does not block this pathway.

(NSAIDs: nonsteroidal anti-inflammatory drugs; PGE2: prostaglandin E2)

TABLE 1.1: Role of other cells in the late phase of urticaria.	
Cells	**Released mediators**
Eosinophils	Major basic protein, eosinophil cationic protein
Basophil	Histamine and leukotrienes
PMNs	No specific role although found in increased number in the lesions
T helper lymphocyte	IL-3, TNF-α

(IL-3: interleukin-3; PMN: polymorphonuclear; TNF-α: tumor necrosis factor-alpha)

Stimuli for mast cell degranulation
- *Allergen*: By cross linking of high affinity IgE receptor
- *Functional autoantibody*: Presence of anti-FcεRIα and anti-IgE
- *Complement induced*: C5a acts as a stimulus for mast cell histamine release
- *Direct mast cell liberators*: Drugs such as opiates and polymyxin B

Nonhistaminergic

- Stimulation of Hageman factor XII activates the intrinsic coagulation system, generation of plasmin, and production of bradykinin.
- There is a complex interconnecting system of feedback loops involving the C1 esterase inhibitor which has an inhibitory influence on the complement, kallikrein, coagulation, and fibrinolytic system.
- The bradykinin which is generated by the action of kallikrein on kininogen appears to be the primary mediators of hereditary angioedema. Whereas the angiotensin-converting enzymes inhibitors (ACEIs) result in accumulation of kinin and lead to angioedema without wheals.

To summarize the pathogenesis of chronic urticaria, a multifactorial model has been put forward
- The lower threshold for urticaria in some persons is due to enhance mast cell releasability.
- This in turn is due to presence of functional autoantibodies, dietary pseudoallergens, stress, viral infection, drugs, and other unknown intrinsic factors.
- The severity of illness may be influenced by frequency, severity and number of aggravating factors that the patient is exposed to simultaneously.

Classification

A. Spontaneous:
- Acute urticaria
- Chronic urticaria

B. Inducible:
- Dermographism
- Cholinergic urticaria
- Contact urticaria
- Cold contact urticaria
- Delayed pressure urticaria
- Heat contact urticaria
- Solar urticaria
- Vibratory urticaria
- Aquagenic urticaria
- Exercise-induced urticaria/angioedema

Urticarial syndrome: Diseases related to urticaria for historical reasons and syndromes that present with hives and/or angioedema—
- Maculopapular cutaneous mastocytosis (urticaria pigmentosa)
- Urticarial vasculitis
- Bradykinin-mediated angioedema (e.g., HAE)
- Exercise-induced anaphylaxis
- Cryopyrin-associated periodic syndromes [(CAPS); urticarial rash, recurrent fever attacks, arthralgia or arthritis, eye inflammation, fatigue, and headaches], i.e., familial cold autoinflammatory syndrome [(FCAS), Muckle–Wells syndrome (MWS), or neonatal onset multisystem inflammatory disease (NOMID)]
- Schnitzler's syndrome (recurrent urticarial rash and monoclonal gammopathy, recurrent fever attacks, bone and muscle pain, arthralgia or arthritis, and lymphadenopathy)
- Gleich's syndrome (episodic angioedema with eosinophilia)
- Well's syndrome (granulomatous dermatitis with eosinophilia)

These diseases and syndromes are related to urticaria: (1) because they present with wheals, angioedema, or both and/or (2) because of historical reasons.
- Chronic Urticaria are of two types: Chronic spontaneous urticaria (CSU) and chronic inducible urticaria (CINDU) **(Fig. 1.9)**
- In some cases, patients may have more than one subtype of urticaria (CSU with CINDU) or overlapping subtypes of CINDU

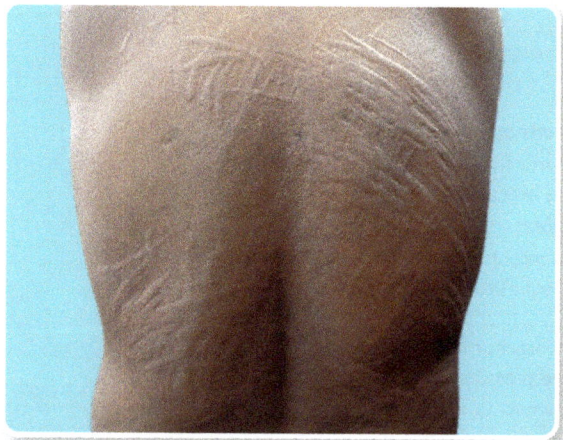

Fig. 1.9: Dermographism on the back.

Quality of Life

- Urticaria is a disease which has severe social, physical, and emotional impact on individual.
- It has a detrimental effect on both objective functioning and subjective wellbeing.
- The tool most widely used to assess the QoL is chronic urticaria quality of life questionnaire (CU-QoL).
- Questionnaire is also developed for angioedema patients.
- Impairment of QoL due to chronic urticaria has been shown to be equal in magnitude to that experienced by patients with triple coronary artery disease awaiting bypass surgery.
- Chronic urticaria is a source of significant economic cost due to absenteeism and cost of medications.
- The impact of chronic urticaria on patient's quality of life (QoL) is similar or greater than that of other chronic skin conditions that cause severe impairment, such as psoriasis and atopic dermatitis.

Clinical Features

Acute Urticaria (Figs. 1.10 to 1.12)

- Spontaneous appearance of wheal and angioedema which lasts less than 6 weeks.

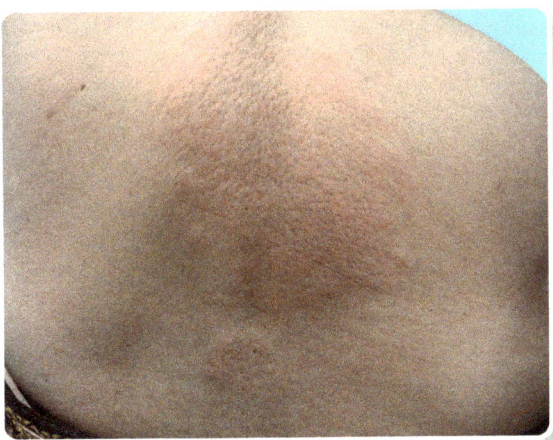

Fig. 1.10: Acute urticaria on the back.

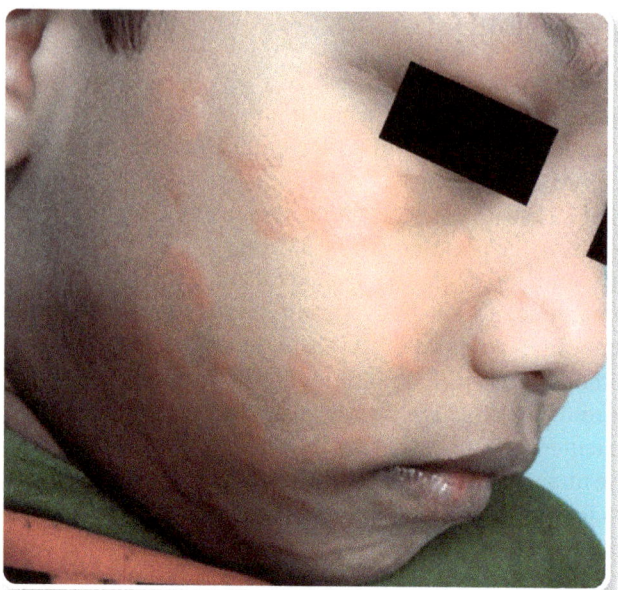

Fig. 1.11: Acute urticaria in a child (postviral).

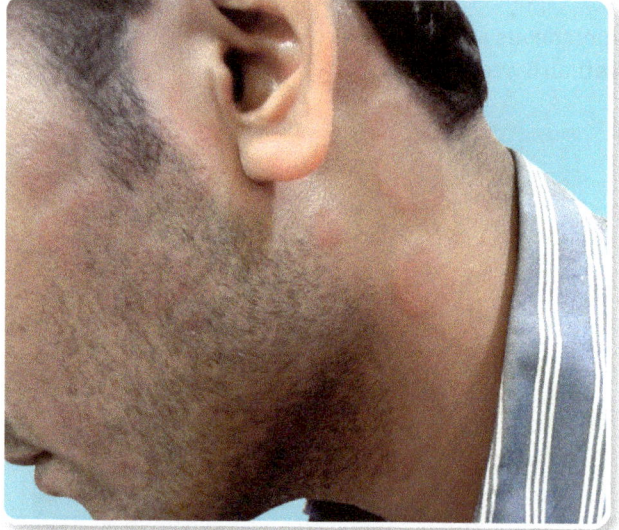

Fig. 1.12: Acute urticaria in an adult male (drug-induced).

TABLE 1.2: Types of acute urticaria.	
Severity of urticaria	**% area affected**
Mild	<10%
Moderate	10–50%
Severe	>50% of systemic affection

- Life time prevalence estimated to be around 15-20%.
- The prevalence of acute urticaria is higher in people with atopic disease, such as hay fever, allergic asthma, and atopic dermatitis.
- It is characterized by discrete scattered wheals size usually larger than 1 cm.
- Angioedema associated in 5% of patients.
- Depending on the body area affected, severity of the disease can be categorized as shown in **Table 1.2**.

Systemic symptoms associated with acute urticaria:
- Shortness of breath
- Dizziness
- Headache
- Nausea
- Diarrhea

Triggering factors of acute urticaria:
- Acute viral upper respiratory tract infection (most common in children)
- Foods and food additives (most common in children), most frequent offender being cow's milk
- Drugs—mainly penicillin and NSAIDs (IgE mediated). Among the NSAIDs, aspirin has the highest propensity to trigger acute urticaria.

Diagnosis:
- Identification of any trigger such as prior infection or drug intake
- Prick test
- Oral provocation tests

(In case of NSAIDs, these tests are not helpful owing to the pseudoallergenic nature of these drug reactions.)

Prognosis:
- Acute urticaria is mostly self-limited in >99% patients.
- Progression to chronic urticaria is rare.

Chronic Urticaria (Fig. 1.13)
- Chronic urticaria is characterized by rapid and noninduced appearance of wheals with or without angioedema, which are usually short-lived.
- Wheals usually last for several hours but angioedema lasts for several days.
- Disease is episodic in nature, with disease period varying from few days to months.
- Peak age is 20–60 years, female commonly affected than male.
- Associated itching or burning
- Mast cells activation is the primary event triggering the disease process

Clinical features:
- About 50% of CU patients have wheals and angioedema together.
- About 40% patients show only wheal and 10% show only angioedema.
- Wheals most commonly develop in the evening hours.

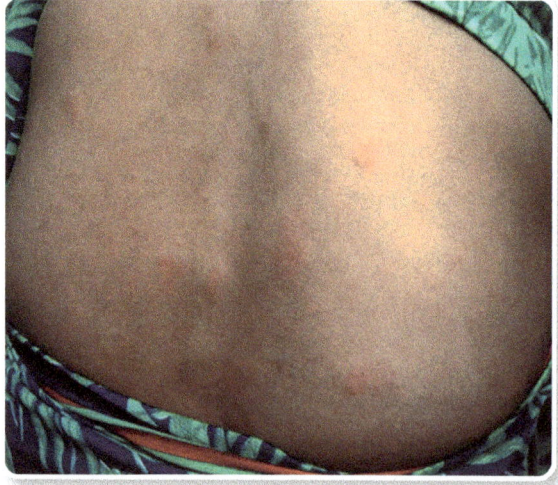

Fig. 1.13: Chronic spontaneous urticaria in a lady.

- Symptoms usually episodic with symptoms-free period ranging from several days to several months.
- Mean duration of disease is 4 years.
- In 50% cases, there is spontaneous remission within 10 years.

> **Extracutaneous features of chronic urticaria**
> - Fever
> - Headache
> - Joint pain
> - Indigestion
> - Diarrhea

Triggering factors of chronic spontaneous urticaria:
- *Autoreactivity*:
  - About 40% of chronic urticaria patients have mast cell activating factors.
  - In only about 20% cases, these factors are anti-IgE or anti-IgE receptor antibody (FcεRI).
  - CU due to autoreactivity is readily detected by autologous serum skin test.
- *Infection*:
  - *Bacterial infection*:
    - Helicobacter pylori gastritis
    - Upper respiratory tract infection by Group A *Streptococci*
  - *Viral infections*:
    - Hepatitis A and B
  - *Parasitic infection*:
    - Toxocara canis
    - Giardia lamblia
    - Blastocystis hominis
  - *Fungal*:
    - Intestinal candidiasis

  (Toll-like receptors present on mast cells functioning as sensors for bacteria, virus and parasites are likely to play an important role in mediating urticarial lesions.)
- *Food intolerance*:
  - Nonallergic dose dependent delayed hypersensitivity to food pseudoallergens, such as:
    - Food colorants
    - Taste intensifiers

- Preservatives
- Naturally occurring substances (fruits, vegetables, and spices)
- Aromatic compounds
- Biogenic amines
- Salicylic acids
(Diagnosed by oral challenge tests with pseudoallergens)
- *Chronic inflammatory process*:
    - Gastritis
    - Reflux esophagitis
    - Chronic cholecystitis
    - Autoimmune disease, such as systemic lupus erythematosus
- *Nonspecific triggers*:
    - Physical exertion
    - Stress

> **Type I allergy**
> - *Rare*: With daily or almost daily symptom
> - *Important*: With intermittent symptoms

> **Psudoallergic to NSAIDs food or food additives**
> - More relevant for CSU with daily symptoms
> - Certain true food allergies can mimic chronic urticaria. This may occur in allergies to food containing omega-5 gliadin, lipid transfer protein (LPT), or galactose-alpha-1,3-galactose

Recognized association of chronic urticaria:
- *Angioedema*: Occurs in 40–80% of patients, mainly affecting eyelids, lips, and tongue.
- *Physical urticaria*: Usually symptomatic dermographism or delayed-pressure urticarial occurs in about 50%.
- *Functional thyroid disease*: Can be associated with both hyper- and hypothyroidism in about 20%. Hashimoto's disease is found in 15% patients.

> **Predictors of disease duration of chronic urticaria**
> - Disease severity at diagnosis
> - Angioedema with or without urticaria
> - Concurrent chronic inducible urticaria (CINDU) with a physical cause
> - Positive autologous serum skin test (ASST)

> **Comorbidities of chronic spontaneous urticaria (CSU)**
> - Depression/anxiety
> - Autoimmune diseases
> - Thyroid dysfunction
> - Metabolic diseases
> - Atopic disorders
> - *H. pylori* gastritis

Autoimmune Urticaria

An autoimmune process is causative in some patients with chronic urticaria referred to as *autoimmune urticaria*.

- About 25–50% of patients of chronic urticaria have complement activating IgG1 and IgG3 autoantibodies against high affinity IgE receptor (FcεR1) or less commonly against IgE receptor.
- These autoantibodies dimerize IgE receptors expressed on dermal mast cells leading to complement activation (C5a) and dermal mast cell activation. No hypocomplementemia associated.
- These autoantibodies have an association with *HLA DRB1*04 and HLA DQB1*0302* (also associated with autoimmune disease).
- Presence of autoantibodies commonly associated with anti-thyroid antibodies.
- Basophils of patients with chronic urticaria are hyporesponsive to circulating anti-IgE antibody.
- Cases of autoimmune urticaria are clinically and histologically indistinguishable from ordinary urticaria.
- These cases tend to run a more aggressive and treatment-resistant course.
- Histologically, increased number of neutrophils and eosinophils, if any, is suggestive, but not confirmatory.

> **Diagnosis of autoimmune urticaria (Fig. 1.14)**
> - Clinically suspected if the response to regular antihistamine is poor
> - Demonstration of antithyroid antibodies suggestive
> - Autologous serum skin test: To be discussed in details in investigation section
> - In vitro testing consists of demonstrating the ability of patient's serum to activate donor basophils.

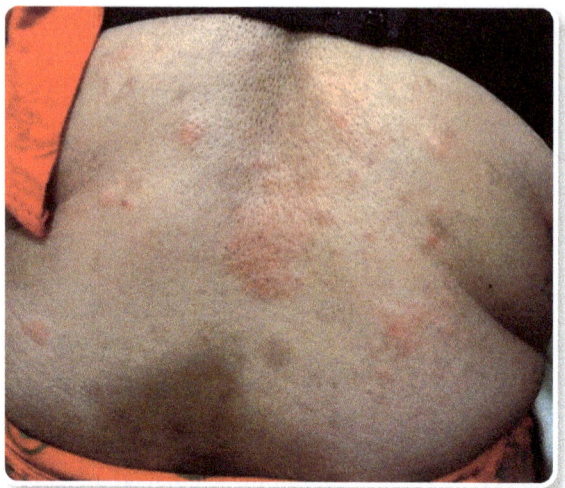

Fig. 1.14: Autoimmune urticaria in a lady.

Autoimmunity versus autoreactivity
- Autoantibodies against IgE or IgE receptor (FcεRI) = Autoimmunity (40% of CU)
- Autologous serum skin test (ASST) + but no autoantibodies = Autoreactivity (80% of CU)
- (Circulating factors for "nonautoimmune" CU with autoreactivity = Not known)

Symptomatic Dermographism

- It is most common form of dermographism where patients complains bouts of itching triggered by a frictional stimuli.
- It can be seen alone or in combination with CSU.
- Commonly encountered physical urticarial, which is frequently overlooked.

Triggering factor:
- Movement of clothing or jewelry on the skin, straps of watches, belts, or elastic tops of socks
- Even touching or rubbing eyes can elicit a response.
- Even a power shower or toweling dry may cause whealing.

Clinical features:
- Onset within minutes and patient complains of generalized itching and red wheals.
- Wheals are polymorphic varying from linear or oblong shape to patchy papular erythema, which can all occur simultaneously.

- Usually take the shape of stimulus applied.
- Mucous membrane is not affected and angioedema is rare.
- The duration is maximum up to 1 hour and disease intensifies in the evening.

Symptomatic dermographism (Figs. 1.15 and 1.16): Short-lived lesions may be found in patients of—
- Mastocytosis
- Scabies
- Bacterial and fungal infections
- Penicillin reactions
- Insect bite hypersensitivity
- Tattoo marks

Other forms of dermographism
- *Physiological dermographism*: There is an asymptomatic wheal and flare, which occurs in 5% of normal population
- *Red dermographism*: A superficial trauma, such as scratching or rubbing evokes an erythematous band with whealing
- *Black dermographism*: Black discoloration of skin occurring after contact with certain metallic objects
- *White dermographism*: This is a blanching response due to capillary vasoconstriction after stroking the skin, seen commonly in atopics.
- *Cholinergic dermographism*: Wheals of cholinergic urticaria appear on stroking the skin.
- *Delayed dermographism*: Delayed pressure urticaria like lesions developing to a frictional stimulus

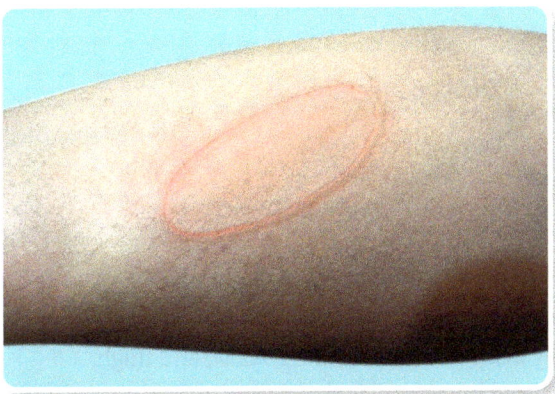

Fig. 1.15: Symptomatic dermographism in a young adult.

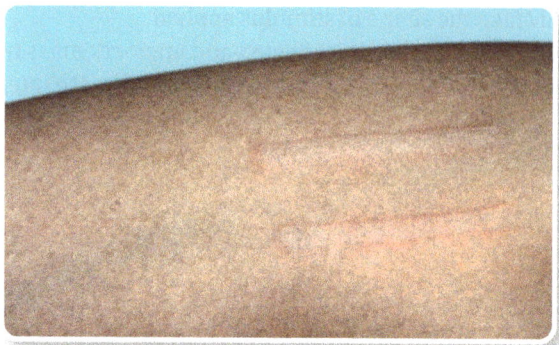

Fig. 1.16: Dermographism in an adult.

> **Diagnosis**
> - Lesions can be reproduced by lightly stroking the upper back with a tongue depressor. A positive response will be visible in 5–10 minutes. A combination of itch, wheal, and flare confirms the diagnosis.
> - A calibrated spring-loaded dermographometer applying different pressures (20–60 g/mm^2) can be used, which enables simultaneous threshold testing
> - Fric test, which consists of six tips stroked over the skin also determines provocation thresholds

Delayed Pressure Urticaria

- There is a delayed response to persistent pressure on skin.
- Suspected in patients who are unresponsive to antihistamines.
- Concurrent with chronic spontaneous urticarial in 40% of cases.
- A sustained pressure stimulus when applied to the skin produces a whealing response, which appears between 30 minutes and 6 hours.

> **Triggering factors**
> - Tight clothing, tight shoes, seatbelt, carrying bags and walking, jogging
> - Sitting on hard chairs produces lesions on buttocks and back of thigh
> - Carrying heavy weights may lead to hand swelling, whereas walking and jogging lead to feet swelling.

Clinical features:
- Painful or itchy erythematous plaques and nodules appear mainly distributed in shoulder, waist, and thigh.
- Swelling of hands and feet can occur.

- Lesions comprise edematous erythematous plaques and nodules and are painful rather than itchy.
- Lesions are deeper than lesions of ordinary urticaria and may persist for a period of 48 hours.
- Associated rarely with arthralgia, malaise, and rigors.

> *Diagnosis:*
> - Histology shows more deeper involvement up to subcutaneous fat with a pronounced cellular infiltrate than other form of urticaria.
>   - Earlier lesions (<5 hours) show a preponderance of neutrophils and eosinophils.
>   - Late lesions (>12 hours) show a preponderance of lymphocytes.
> - Lesions of delayed pressure urticaria (DPU) can be reproduced by pressure, and a positive pressure test can be elicited by:
>   - When a 15 lb weight suspended from forearm for 15 minutes and the lesions are produced within 30 minutes to 6 hours
>   - Application of metal rods of different weights can be applied on thighs or back. With the convex end diameter of the rods of 1.5 cm weights of 2.5 or 4.5 kg applied for 20 and 15 minutes respectively. In patients of DPU, an indurated wheal occurs 6 hour later at the application site.
>   - Dermographometer set at a pressure of 100 g/mm^2 pressed against back for 70 seconds and inspected 6 hours later
> - Laboratory parameters which may be altered during attack include:
>   - – Raised erythrocyte sedimentation rate (ESR)
>   - – Neutrophil leukocytosis
>   - – Elevated alpha-1 antitrypsin level

- DPU is a disease of varying severity combined with episodes of remissions and exacerbations over weeks and months.
- May be concurrent with chronic spontaneous urticarial and dermographism.
- Lifestyle modification such as wearing loose clothing, soft slightly loose shoes is equally important to pharmacological management **(Figs. 1.17 and 1.18)**.

Heat and Cold Urticaria

- Cold urticaria is a commonly encountered subtype of physical urticaria with prevalence of 0.5% in general population with highest prevalence in young adults.
- Disease is of variable severity and stimulation temperatures vary widely among individuals.

- Sometimes generalized urticaria can be elicited even at room temperature.
- Severe forms can sometimes be accompanied by hypotension and fainting.
- Heat urticaria resembles cold urticaria but the eliciting stimulus is contact with objects having temperatures above normal skin temperature.

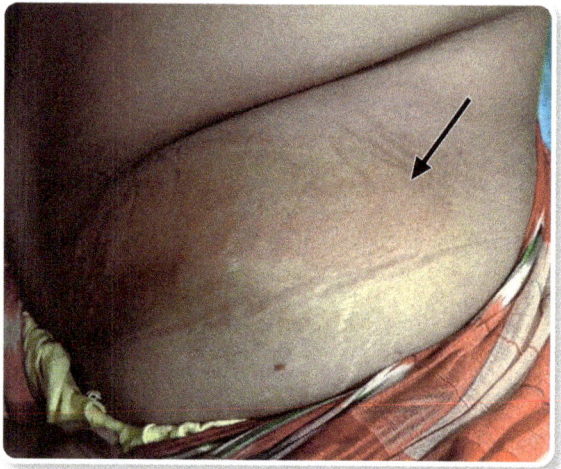

Fig. 1.17: Delayed pressure urticaria in a lady at her waistline by petticoat's pressure.

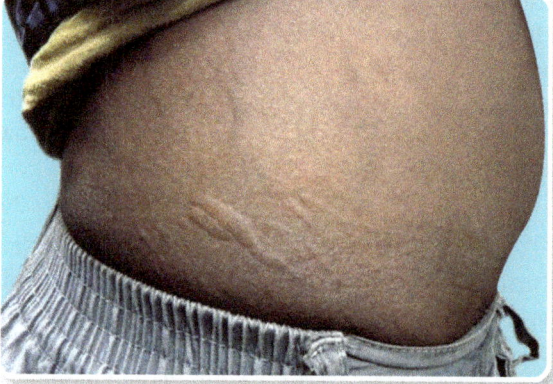

Fig. 1.18: Delayed pressure urticaria along waistline in a male.

Types of cold urticaria (based on cold stimulation test):
- Positive cold stimulation test
- Negative cold stimulation test

Negative cold stimulation test
- Delayed cold urticaria:
  - Whealing takes place hours after stimulation
- Cold dependent dermographism:
  - Lesions elicited by stroking precooled skin
- Systemic atypical acquired cold urticaria:
  - Only a specific stimulus, (e.g., cold wind) can elicit whealing
- Cold induced cholinergic urticaria:
  - Lesions elicited when exercising in cold environment
- Familial cold autoinflammatory syndrome:
  - Urticaria with conjunctivitis, fever, deafness, and lymphadenopathy

---

Positive cold stimulation test
- Primary cold urticaria
- *Secondary cold urticaria*:
  - Infection, e.g., infectious mononucleosis, bacterial infections
  - Drugs
  - Cryoglobulinemia
  - Vasculitis
  - Malignancies

Pathogenesis:
- Most important cell in pathogenesis of cold urticaria is *mast cell* which gets activated on cooling below threshold liberating vasoactive mediators.
- Neutrophils, eosinophils, and platelets also suggested to play a role.
- About 30-40% patients of cold urticarial have autoantibodies against IgE or against high affinity receptor for IgE.
- Mediators are mainly histamine, prostaglandin D2, and platelet activating factor.
- But the mechanism of heat urticaria is unclear.

Clinical features **(Fig. 1.19)**:
- Heat and cold urticaria can be *triggered* by:
  - Exposure to cold or warm environments

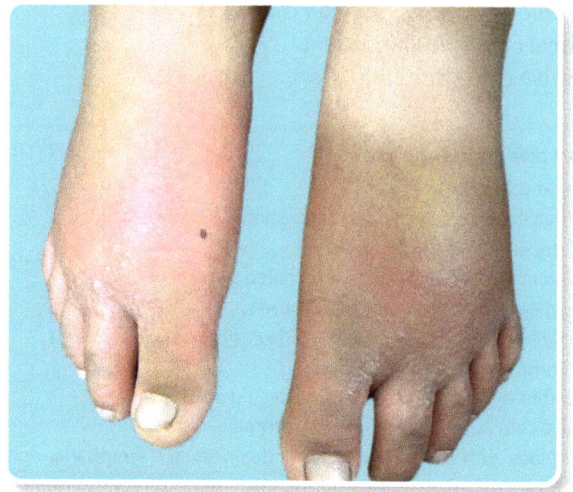

Fig. 1.19: Cold urticaria in a child of 10 years.

- ○ Ingestion of cold or warm food and beverages
- ○ Handling of cold or warm objects
- ○ Aquatic activities
- Major symptoms are immediate development of pruritic wheals and/or angioedema which are typically *nonpseudopodic*.
- Wheals or angioedema may be localized or generalized.
- Exposure of cold to upper aerodigestive tract may lead to swelling of lips, tongue, pharynx, or larynx and even lead to syncope.
- *Severity depends on two factors*:
  i. Area of skin involved
  ii. Difference between temperature of stimulus and patients threshold

---

Types of cold urticaria
Based on cold urticaria severity, it can be classified into:
- Type 1: Localized urticaria at site of exposure (most common)
- Type 2: Generalized urticaria
- Type 3: Severe generalized urticaria with hypotension

- It may be dangerous when attacks occur during aquatic activities as it may lead to drowning.

Diagnosis:
- Cold *stimulation test* is done by placing melting ice cube in thin polythene on volar aspect of forearm for 5 minutes and observing the wheal appearing after minutes of removal of stimulus (the ice should be melting to avoid skin damage at temperature <0°C and should be placed in a plastic bag to avoid confusion with aquagenic urticaria).
- *Temperature test* is a new method to determine the patient's threshold temperature by exposure of the skin to the thermal elements with defined temperatures to assess the stimulation temperature and time.

Temperature test using testing kits can be used to determine the critical temperature thresholds for cold contact urticaria and the more rare heat contact urticaria.
- Differential leukocyte count
- ESR and C-reactive protein (CRP)
- Autologous serum skin test to evaluate the autoimmunity
- Antinuclear antibody
- Infectious mononucleosis and syphilis serology
- Total complement level
- Cryoglobulin levels

Prognosis:
- Prolonged course with mean disease duration exceeding 10 years.
- Apart from the pharmacological treatment tolerance induction plays an important role in desensitization.

Solar Urticaria (Fig. 1.20)
- It is characterized by whealing response of skin which develops between 5 and 10 minute of exposure to visible light or UV light.
- Itching or burning sensation commonly associated with wheals.
- Lesions usually last for few hours and affect mainly covered body areas than the face and hands.
- Usually occurs in between second and fourth decade and more prevalent in females.
- It may be associated with systemic symptoms such as headache, nausea, wheezing, dyspnea, etc.
- It occurs usually between spring and autumn.

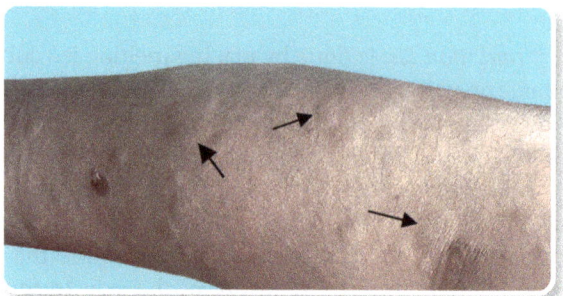

Fig. 1.20: Solar urticarial on forearm in a 43-year-old lady.

Solar urticaria: Associations—
- Atopy
- Polymorphic light eruption
- Chronic actinic dermatitis
- SLE
- Other physical urticaria

Pathogenesis:
- Degranulation of mast cells releasing histamine among other mediators plays an important role in whealing response.
- Eosinophils and neutrophils also participate in pathogenesis.
- Wheals are caused by exposure to specific wavelength of light, called action spectra which include visible light, UVA, and UVB.
- Autologous photoallergens play an important role in the pathogenesis.
- Patients with action spectrum 400–500 nm have a photoallergen of molecular weight 25–45 kd, while those with action spectrum 330–520 nm have photoallergen of molecular weight 300–1,000 kd.
- Two types of photoallergens identified:
  i. Patient-specific photoallergen
  ii. Nonspecific photoallergens, i.e., found universally in all persons
- Suspected photoallergens include:
  ○ Porphyrin—responsible for solar urticaria in patients of erythropoietic porphyria and porphyria cutanea tarda.
  ○ Drugs such as tetracycline, chlorpromazine, and progesterone
  ○ Chemicals such as coal tar and pitch

Diagnosis:
- Provocation test using a solar simulator to apply UVA (up to 6 J/cm^2) and UVB (up to 0.06 J/cm^2) or a projector to apply visible light (to exclude other causes) to patches of skin on the buttocks. An urticarial response is usually visible within 10 minutes.

Cholinergic Urticaria (Fig. 1.21)
- Cholinergic urticaria is characterized by small short-lived wheals occurring after a *rise in the core temperature*.
- Most frequently occurs in young adults with no sex predilection.
- Peak prevalence seen in between 10 and 30 years of age.

Pathogenesis
- Mast cell degranulation and histamine release has been implicated.
- Role of acetylcholine released from local sympathetic nerve ending has been speculated.
- Type-1 hypersensitivity reaction to sweat has been suggested but not substantiated.

Clinical features: Triggers of cholinergic urticaria:
- Activities which increase core body temperature such as:
  - Exercise to the point of sweating
  - Emotion
  - Eating hot and spicy food

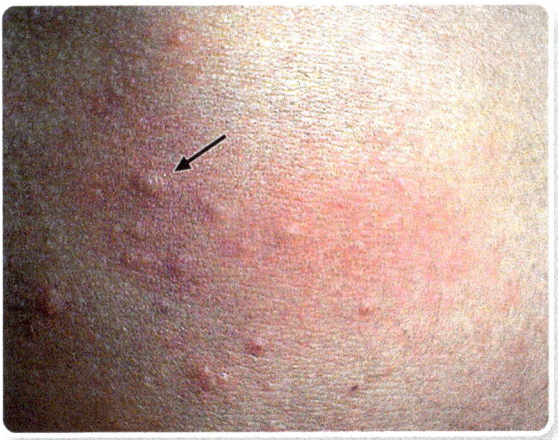

Fig. 1.21: Cholinergic urticaria.

- Exposure to high ambient temperature
- Hot shower
• Patients undergoing hemodialysis
  - Extremely itchy wheals which are characteristically small (2-3 mm) having a large surrounding flare.
  - Multiple wheals may coalesce to form plaques.
  - Commonly found on upper trunk and proximal limbs.

Associated systemic symptoms include
- Dizziness
- Flushing
- Headache
- Abdominal pain
- Nausea and diarrhea
- Wheezing and breathlessness
- Hypotension

Disease associations of cholinergic urticaria:
- Chronic spontaneous urticaria
- Cold urticaria
- Dermographism

Diagnosis:
- Lesions elicited by exercising the patient to the point of sweating
- Passive warming by hot bath test can be done to reproduce the lesions where patient is almost immersed in a bath at 42°C for 15 minutes
- False negative results may be found in:
  - If the patient is in refractory period after an attack
  - Already on treatment, hence treatment should be withdrawn before testing.
  - Patients should be carefully monitored during testing as anaphylaxis can occur during testing.
- Provocative test includes ergometric testing (use of an exercise machine or physical activity of any description to the point of sweating). If this test is positive it should be followed by bathing at 42°C for 15 minutes to increase body temperature by ≥1°C. A positive exercise test but negative hot bath test indicates exercise-induced urticaria.

Differential diagnosis: To be differentiated from other *cutaneous disorder precipitated by rise in the core temperature*:
- Cholinergic pruritus:
    - Short-lived itching occurs.
- *Exercise-induced anaphylaxis*:
    - Anaphylaxis is precipitated by exercise only, not by other causes of increase core temperature.
- Persisting cholinergic erythema:
    - Multiple monomorphic red itchy macules in a widespread distribution confirmed by observing the persistence of lesions up to 1-2 hours.
- *Cold induced cholinergic urticaria and cholinergic dermographism*: Lesions can be reproduced by reduction of core temperature or by stroking the skin respectively.
- *Localized heat urticaria*: Confirmed by the development of lesions at the site of contact of warm objects against the skin, without any need for rise in core body temperature.
- *Aquagenic urticaria*: Triggered by exposure to water of any temperature, e.g., taking a tepid bath with water at 37°C will trigger aquagenic urticaria but not cholinergic urticaria.
- *Dermographism after bath*:
    - Rubbing of skin during bath may trigger dermographism.
    - Can be confirmed by gentle scratching the skin (pressure <36 g/mm^3).
    - To rule out atopic dermatitis as these patients complain of itching after bath.

Exercise-induced Anaphylaxis

- It is a rare entity where only *physical exertion* can lead to anaphylaxis.
- Exercise-induced anaphylaxis (EIA) is not induced by other passive causes of an increased core temperature not even by sweating. This *distinguishes* it from *cholinergic urticaria*.
- In some cases, ingestion of foods such as wheat, shell fish, apples, peaches or drugs, such as aspirin, play a permissive role in the attack.
- More common in atopics.
- Sex ratio varies among different studies.
- Mast cell degranulation plays an important role during attack.

- Cutaneous symptoms include:
    - Pruritus
    - Wheals (sometimes of cholinergic type)
    - Flushing
    - Angioedema
- Associated systemic features are:
    - Cough, dyspnea, and wheezing
    - Intestinal colic, nausea, diarrhea
    - Headache, vertigo, tinnitus
    - Systemic symptoms may last from 30 minutes to 4 hours, but headache can last up to 72 hours.

> **Food-dependent EIA**
> Two subgroups of patients with food-dependent EIA have been found:
> - One group may have anaphylaxis when exercising in close proximity to ingestion of any type of food, and the another group experiencing anaphylaxis with exercise with prior ingestion of a specific food.

Diagnosis:
- History is sufficient most of the times.
- Lesions can be reproduced by exercising the patient but with proper monitoring with treatment of anaphylaxis available.
- Prick tests or specific IgE measurement to individual food stuff when there is positive challenge.

Vibratory Urticaria

- Subjects with vibratory angioedema experience pruritus and swelling with exposure of the skin to a vibratory stimulus.
- This condition can be familial.
- Vibratory angioedema can be confirmed by demonstrating an exaggerated response after exposure of the skin to a vortex mixer (1,000 rpm) for 10 minutes on the forearm.

Contact Urticaria

- It is defined as the wheals that appear following contact of exogenous substances with the skin **(Figs. 1.22 and 1.23)**.
- This is of two types:
    i. Immunologic contact urticaria/allergic contact urticaria
    ii. Nonimmunologic contact urticaria

> **Immunologic contact urticaria**
> - IgE mediated type 1 hypersensitivity reaction
> - Rapid-acting counterpart of allergic contact dermatitis, although rarely delayed onset is possible
> - Most inducers are protein in nature, but smaller molecules can act as haptens in producing an urticarial reaction
> - Associated with systemic symptoms, hence the term contact urticaria syndrome has been proposed

Immunological contact urticaria: Common inducers—
- Animal products like hair, blood, gelatin, etc. Amniotic fluid is a major problem in veterinarians.
- Plant products mainly latex can trigger allergic reaction in those using latex gloves. Those with latex allergy are also at an increased risk of developing allergic reactions to foods such as bananas and tomatoes.
  - Use of low powder, low latex containing gloves has greatly reduced sensitization rates.
- Food such as banana, tomatoes, onion, garlic, dairy product, fish, etc.
  - Protein contact dermatitis is a type of contact urticaria seen in food handlers who develop itching, erythema, wheals, and dyshidrosiform changes.

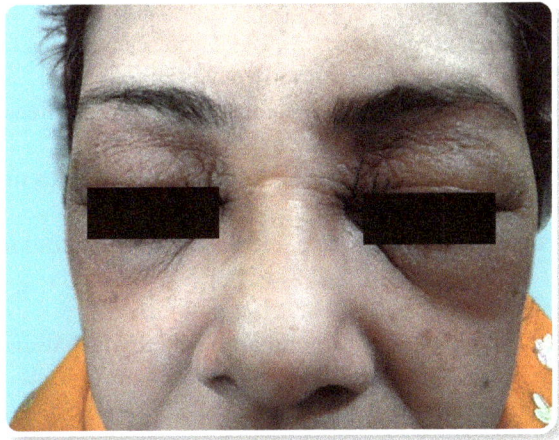

Fig. 1.22: Contact urticaria in a lady from hair dye.

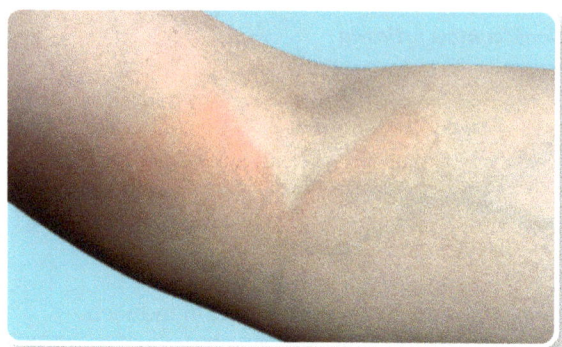

Fig. 1.23: Contact urticaria in a lady from fragrance.

- Intake of offending foods may lead to perioral erythema, tingling, burning and swelling of lips, tongue, oral mucosa.
- Diagnosed by positive skin prick tests and positive RAST
• Contact with medication like phenothiazine, pyrazolone, benzocaine
• *Miscellaneous*: Ammonium persulfate (used as bleaching agents by beauticians), epoxies, and acrylic

> **Nonimmunologic contact urticaria**
> ♦ Can occur on first exposure to an individual who come in contact to the offending agent.
> ♦ Lesions restricted to the site of contact on skin.
> ♦ Lack systemic symptoms.

Nonimmunological contact urticaria: Common triggering factors—
• Plants—stinging nettle (contain toxin in their leaves)
• Animal—caterpillars, jellyfish, mosquito, ants, and fleas
  - Papular urticaria like lesions commonly seen
  - Sometimes, lesions can be found at distant sites mimicking immunologic urticaria.
  - Scabies can present with urticaria due to sensitization to mite.
• *Direct histamine liberators*:
  - Spices for example, mustard, cinnamon
  - Fragrance, for example, cinnamon aldehyde, balsam of Peru
  - Medications, for example, menthol, camphor, benzocaine, alcohol, bacitracin, polymyxin
  - Preservatives, for example, benzoic acid, sorbic acid, formaldehyde

Diagnosis:
- Repeat open application test (ROAT)
- Open patch test (open patch test to be done instead of closed method by Fin chamber as closed one may induce more absorption of allergens that may lead to anaphylaxis)
- Desensitization following controlled exposure, such as repeated wearing of latex gloves
- Prick test (should be done with prior withdrawal of antihistamines for 72 hours. The test should not be performed during acute disease activity)
- In-use challenge prick testing with potential triggers (e.g., fruits, latex gloves, etc.) applied directly to the skin (any provocation test should be conducted with caution and facilities for emergency treatment during provocation should be available).
- Radioallergosorbent test (RAST)

Urticarial Vasculitis (Figs. 1.24 to 1.26)

- *Clinicopathological entity characterized by*:
    - Urticarial papules and plaques usually lasting longer than 24 hours duration
    - Resolving with faint purpura or residual hyperpigmentation
    - Histologically characterized by presence of leukocytoclastic vasculitis in capillaries and postcapillary venules, with or without fibrinoid deposits.
- Prevalence is 5% in general population with female predominance.
- Peak incidence in fourth decade of life
- Deposition of immune complexes appears to trigger the inflammatory cascade.
- *Triggers of urticarial vasculitis include*:
    - Autoimmune connective tissue disease:
        - Sjögren's syndrome
        - Systemic lupus
        - Rheumatoid arthritis
    - Infections:
        - Hepatitis B and C
        - Paraproteinemias
        - Inflammatory bowel disease
        - Serum sickness like drug reaction
        - Idiopathic

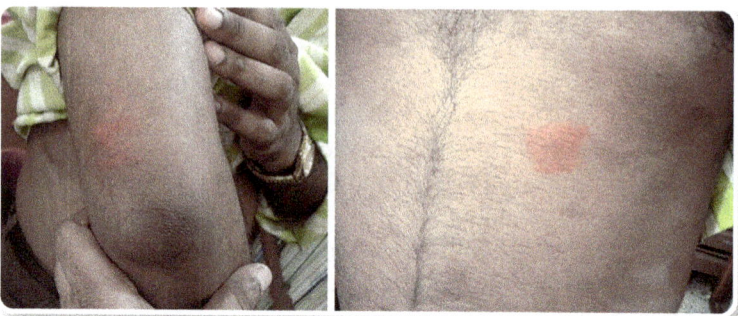

Fig. 1.24: Urticarial vasculitis in a man: Lesion persisting more the 24 hours.

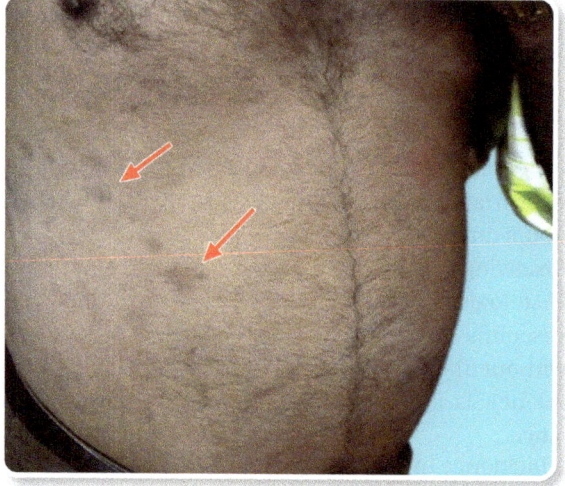

Fig. 1.25: Urticarial vasculitis in a man: posturticarial pigmentation.

Types:
- Normocomplementemic urticarial vasculitis
- Hypocomplementemic urticarial vasculitis
- Hypocomplementemic urticarial vasculitic syndrome (HUVS) when associated with constellation of systemic features
  [IgG autoantibodies to the collagen like region of C1q found commonly in patients of HUVS are also detectable in fair number of patients of systemic lupus erythematosus (SLE) and even more in SLE with glomerulonephritis. Hence, these patients are to be properly followed up.]

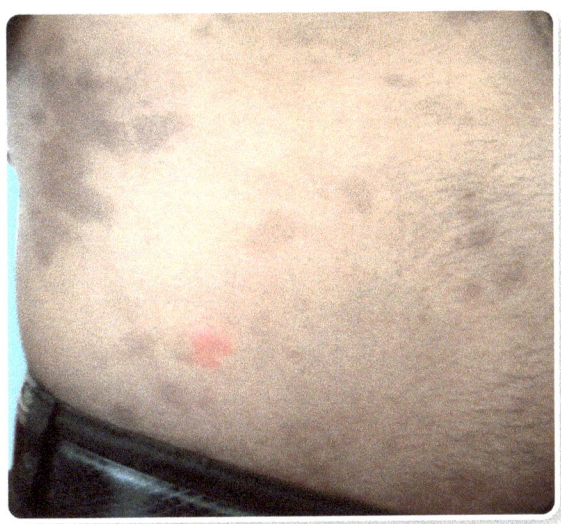

Fig. 1.26: Urticarial vasculitis in another man with posturticarial pigmentation.

Clinical features
- Urticarial papules and plaque which are burning and tender rather than pruritic.
- Angioedema seen in 42% cases
- Giant lesions less common
- Lesions common in areas subject to pressure
- Lesions resolve with residual purpura or hyperpigmentation.
- Rarely, associated with livedo reticularis, erythema multiforme, or bullae

Systemic features
- Musculoskeletal involvement:
  - Transient and migratory peripheral arthralgia
  - Jaccoud's arthropathy (patients at increased risk of valvular heart disease)
- Renal involvement:
  - Proteinuria and microscopic hematuria
  - Mesangial proliferative glomerulonephritis
  - Interstitial nephritis
- Pulmonary involvement:
  - Dyspnea and cough
  - Hemoptysis

- Pleuritis
- Emphysema and chronic obstructive pulmonary disease (COPD)
* Gastrointestinal involvement:
  - Abdominal pain
  - Nausea and vomiting
  - Diarrhea
* Ophthalmological involvement:
  - Conjunctivitis
  - Episcleritis
  - Uveitis and iritis
* Miscellaneous:
  - Pericarditis and pericardial effusion
  - Valvular heart disease
  - Pseudotumor cerebri
  - Peripheral neuropathy
  - Raynaud's phenomenon

> **Urticarial vasculitic lesions could sometimes be**
> - Short lasting, staying less than 24 hours, and similar to CU. Thus urticarial vasculitis cannot be completely excluded based on the history of lesions duration less than 24 hours. Whenever, suspected diagnosis of urticarial vasculitis should be confirmed by a biopsy showing the presence of leukocytoclastic vasculitis.

Investigations:
* Skin biopsy: Shows leukocytoclastic vasculitis with fibrinoid necrosis of postcapillary venules
* Direct immunofluorescence: Shows presence of immunoglobulins, compliments and fibrin within vessel walls
* Complete hemogram
* Shows elevation of ESR and C-reactive protein
* Viral screen: For hepatitis A and B
* Plasma protein electrophoresis
* ANF, anti-Ro, and rheumatoid factor
* Chest X-ray, ECG, and echocardiogram
* Compliment screen
* Measurement of serum C1q, C3, C4, and CH50

Differential Diagnosis

- *Papular urticaria*: Commonly seen in children on exposed area as tiny urticarial lesions with central puncta induced by insect bites. Atopics are more prone **(Fig. 1.27)**.
- *Erythema multiforme*: May resemble urticaria usually showing targetoid lesions usually on acral areas **(Fig. 1.28)**.
- *Polymorphous light eruption*: Differs from solar urticaria in that the onset usually occurs minutes to hours after sunlight exposure and the eruption, which occurs in different forms, including papules, papulovesicles, and plaques, lasts for days compared with solar urticaria, which is short-lived between exposures.
- *Polymorphic eruption of pregnancy (pruritic urticarial papules and plaques of pregnancy or PUPPP)*: Urticaria-like dermatoses can occur at various stages of pregnancy.
- *Autoimmune progesterone-induced dermatitis*: Women presenting with cyclical urticaria related to menstruation.
- *Recall urticaria*: Urticaria is observed at the site of a previous sting or injection after re-exposure to the same inciting factor.
- *Hypereosinophilic syndrome*: Peripheral total eosinophil count exceeds 1,500/mL in the absence of other causes for peripheral eosinophilia.

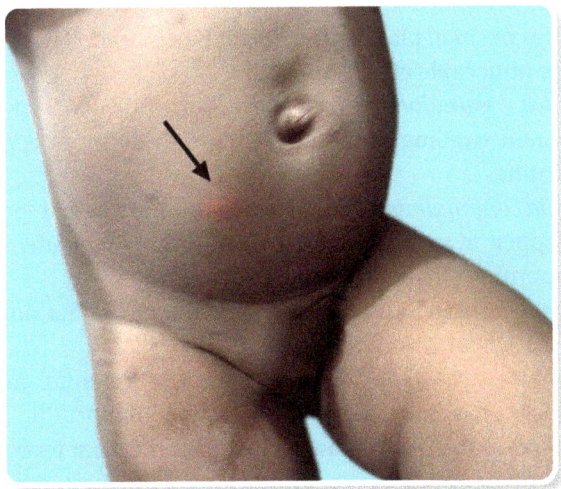

Fig. 1.27: Papular urticaria in a child.

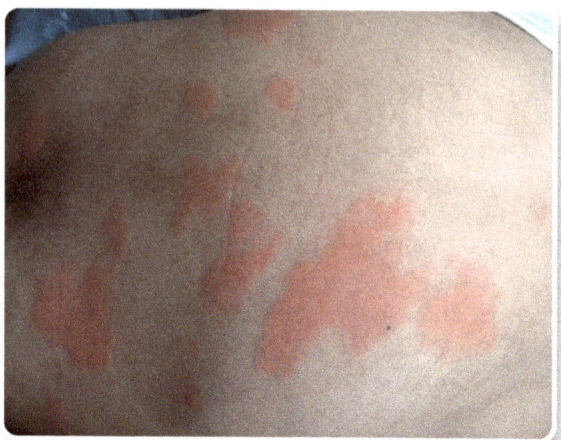

Fig. 1.28: Erythema multiforme on back.

- *Cutaneous mast cell disorders*: Present with urticaria-like lesions include urticaria pigmentosa, mastocytomas, and telangiectasia macularis eruptiva perstans. Apart from urticaria and angioedema, patients usually have additional systemic symptoms.
- *Bullous pemphigoid*: This can present initially with urticaria-like papules or small plaques that might be excoriated by the patient before noticeable blistering occurs.
- *Cheilitis granulomatosa (Melkersson–Rosenthal syndrome)*: Persistent swelling of the lips without evidence of eczematous dermatitis.
- *Thyroid ophthalmopathy*: Swelling of the medial portion of the upper eyes, a sign of thyroid ophthalmopathy, may be misinterpreted as angioedema.
- *Gleich syndrome*: Episodic attacks of angioedema and weight gain along with eosinophilia.
- *Schnitzler syndrome*: Caused by an IgM or more rarely IgG monoclonal gammopathy present with nonpruritic urticaria (that spares the face), bone pain, and intermittent fever.

Diagnosis of Acute Urticaria

- Acute urticaria and angioedema more frequently associated with identifiable conditions
- Acute urticaria and angioedema will usually resolve spontaneously, laboratory evaluation for chronic illness not required unless supported by the clinical history or physical examination.
- Empiric elimination diets (not guided by history and testing) are not recommended.
- Some cases of acute urticaria are caused by viral or other infectious illnesses. However, extensive evaluation for specific viral pathogens or antiviral therapy is not indicated unless suggested by the clinical history.
- Skin testing or immunoassays to identify specific triggers for acute urticaria and angioedema can be helpful if an allergic cause is suggested by history.
  (Skin testing is to be done after the resolution of acute urticaria and after withdrawal of antihistamines or by serologic testing in the presence of significant dermatographism.)

Diagnosis of Chronic Urticaria

- Because of the heterogeneity of the disease initial evaluation should start with history and routine physical examination.
- Specific laboratory test and provocation test should be performed if there are suggestive features in history.
- Invasive and costly investigations are to be strongly discouraged.
- Infectious cause should be considered in urticaria associated with ear, nose and throat infections, dental infections, and *H. pylori* infections.
- *Anisakis simplex*, a sea fish nematode, is frequently associated with urticarial in population who consume uncooked sea fish.
- Other infections associated with urticaria are *H. pylori, Streptococcus species, Staphylococcus species, Giardia*, hepatitis, etc.
- Ruling out malignancies is warranted only if patient's history is suggestive.

Routine questionnaire for evaluating a case of urticaria includes:
1. Time of onset of disease
2. Frequency/duration of and provoking factors for wheals
3. Diurnal variation
4. Occurrence in relation to weekends, holidays, and foreign travel
5. Shape, size, and distribution of wheals
6. Associated angioedema
7. Associated subjective symptoms of lesions, for example, itch, pain, etc.
8. Family and personal history regarding urticaria, atopy
9. Previous or current allergies, infections, internal diseases, or other possible causes
10. Psychosomatic and psychiatric diseases
11. Surgical implantations and events during surgery, for example after local anesthesia
12. Gastric/intestinal problems
13. Induction by physical agents or exercise
14. Use of drugs (e.g., NSAIDs, injections, immunizations, hormones, laxatives, suppositories, ear and eye drops, and alternative remedies)
15. Observed correlation to food
16. Relationship to the menstrual cycle
17. Smoking habits (especially use of perfumed tobacco products or cannabis)
18. Type of work
19. Hobbies
20. Stress
21. Quality of life related to urticaria and emotional impact
22. Previous therapy and response to therapy
23. Previous diagnostic procedures/results

Duration of chronic inducible urticaria (CINDU)
- Most cases of CINDU last ≤1 hour
  [Exception: Contact urticaria (2 hours) and delayed pressure urticaria (24 hours)]

Recommended tests:

Types	Subtypes	Routine diagnostic tests	Extended diagnostic tests (if history suggests)
Spontaneous urticaria	a. Acute spontaneous urticaria	None	None
	b. Chronic spontaneous urticaria	Differential blood count, ESR, CRP, omission of suspected drugs	Tests for infectious disease, type 1 allergy, functional autoantibodies, thyroid hormones and autoantibodies, skin tests including physical tests, pseudoallergen free diet for 3 weeks, tryptase assay, ASST, lesional skin biopsy
Inducible urticaria	a. Cold urticaria	Cold provocation test	Differential blood count, ESR, CRP, cryoproteins and infectious disease detection
	b. Delayed pressure urticaria	Pressure test **(Fig. 1.29)**	None
	c. Heat urticaria	Heat provocation test	None
	d. Solar urticaria	UV and visible light threshold test	Rule out other photodermatosis
	e. Symptomatic dermographism	Test for dermographism	Differential count, ESR, CRP
	f. Vibratory angioedema	Test with vortex	None
	g. Aquagenic urticaria	Wet clothes at body temperature for 20 minutes	None
	h. Cholinergic urticaria	Exercise and hot bath provocation	None
	i. Contact urticaria	Prick test	None

(ESR: erythrocyte sedimentation rate; CRP: C-reactive protein)

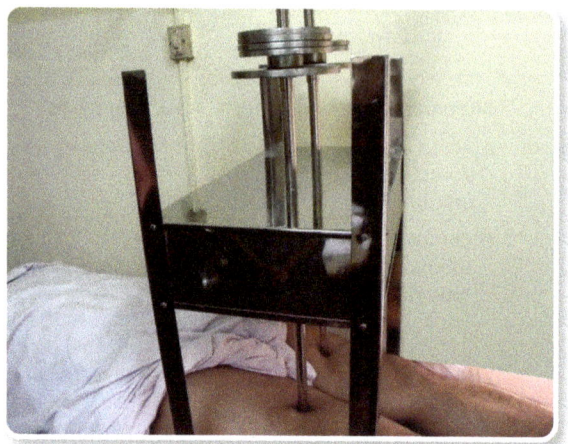

Fig. 1.29: Delayed pressure urticaria detecting instrument.

*Clinical approach in a case of lesions with hives (**Flowchart 1.1**):*

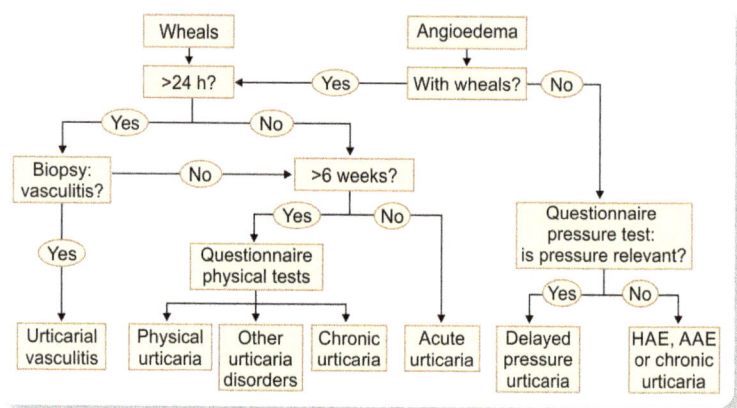

Flowchart 1.1: Algorithm in clinical approach in urticaria.

Test for autoantibodies:

Autoantibody screening
- Autologous serum skin test (ASST)
- Basophil release test

- Currently, the only generally available test to screen for autoantibodies against either IgE or FcεRI (the high affinity receptor) is the autologous serum skin test (ASST), a nonspecific screening test that evaluates the presence of serum histamine-releasing factors of any type, not just histamine-releasing autoantibodies.
- In some countries, a basophil release test is available and may be used, which is a more refined laboratory test that evaluates the in-vitro histamine release from basophils.

Autologous serum skin test (ASST) (Figs. 1.30 and 1.31)

Currently the only available test to screen for autoantibodies is the autologous serum skin test (ASST)

- This is a nonspecific test that evaluates the presence of histamine releasing factor
- It is a very simple, quick test which consists of intradermal injection of patient's own serum with a 0.4 mm needle into the volar aspect of forearm
- Positive control with histamine and negative control with 0.9% saline is also injected 3–5 cm apart
- The reading is taken 30 minutes later and the diameter of the wheal at the test site is measured
- Positive reading means diameter at the test site should be at least 1.5 mm larger than the negative control
- To be performed with utmost care because infections might be transmitted if, by mistake, patients were injected with someone else's serum

---

[Autologous plasma skin test (APST): Higher positive response than ASST. This could be due to coagulation factors enhance vascular permeability or induce mast cell granulation.]

ASST: Limitations—

There are no definitive studies demonstrating that patients with refractory CU and a positive ASST result respond differently to certain medication regimens compared with those patients with CU with a negative ASST result. Current evidence does not support routine performance of ASSTs or autologous plasma skin tests (APST) in patients with CU.

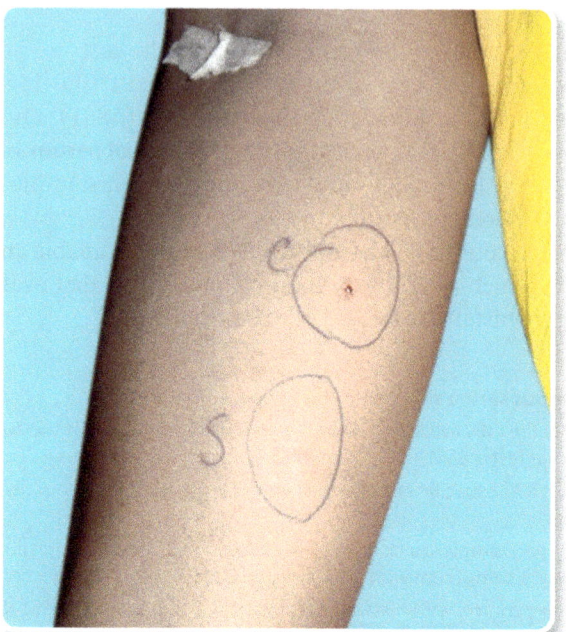

Fig. 1.30: Autologous serum skin test (immediately after).

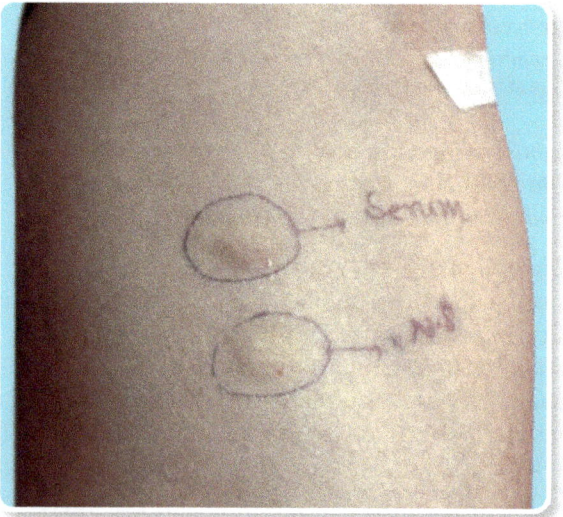

Fig. 1.31: Autologous serum skin test (significantly positive after 30 minutes).

Additional blood tests:

> **Blood tests:**
> - Antinuclear antibody test
> - D-dimer level
> - Blood basophil count

- Antinuclear antibody test can also be considered if the patient history suggests.
- An elevated D-dimer level seen in some CSU patients, who responded to anticoagulation therapy.
- Several groups have noted blood basopenia and that blood basophils exhibit suppressed IgE-receptor-mediated histamine release to anti-IgE. Blood basophils are detected in skin lesions and in nonlesional skin of CSU patients. CSU remission is associated with increases in blood basophil numbers and IgE receptor triggered histamine response.

Tests for physical urticaria:

> **Physical urticaria test:**
> - Cold urticaria: Temperature test
> - Symptomatic dermographism: Dermographometer
> - Delayed pressure urticaria: Modified Illing method and dermographometer (**Fig. 1.32**)
> - Cholinergic urticaria: Ergometer provocation test

- In physical urticaria, the routine diagnosis attempts to identify the subtype by the appropriate physical stimulation tests and to determine trigger thresholds. The latter is important as it allows for assessing disease severity and response to treatment.
- For most types of physical urticaria, no validated tools for provocation testing exist.

Tests for Contact Urticaria

> - Prick test
> - Open patch test

Contact urticaria should be demonstrated with cutaneous provocation tests, for example prick tests or open patch test (**Fig. 1.33**).

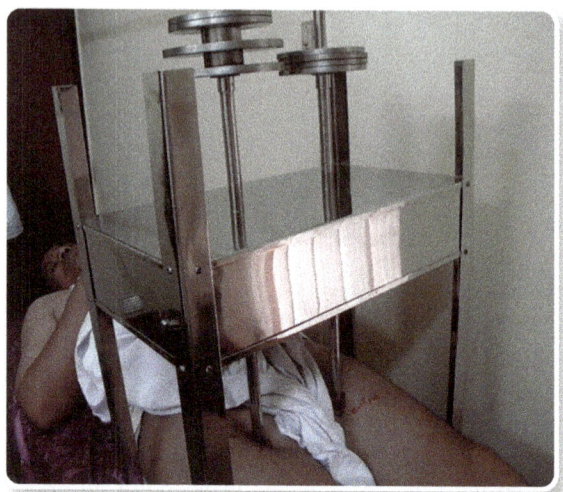

Fig. 1.32: Delayed pressure urticaria: Detection by instrument with different weights (modified Illing method).

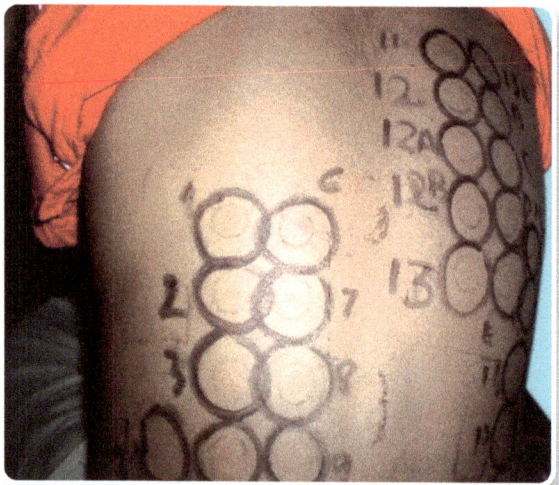

Fig. 1.33: Open patch test in a suspected case of contact urticaria.

- Prick test demands withdrawal of antihistamines for at least 72 hours prior to test.
- Open patch test is justified in contact urticaria as occlusion by Fin chamber may induce increased absorption of allergens that can lead to anaphylaxis.

Diagnosis in Children

> **Urticaria in children:**
> - Acute spontaneous urticaria is common in infants and young children, especially in atopics
> - Triggers include acute viral infection and food (common in infants and young children)
> - Anaphylaxis can happen from food, like milk, egg, peanut, etc.
> - Underlying causes in CSU in child and adults are not much different except in infants.

- Urticaria can occur in all age groups.
- Acute spontaneous urticaria is common in infants and young children, particularly in atopics.
- Triggers include acute viral infection or (more frequently than in older children and adults) ingestion of food such as milk, egg, or peanut, to which the infant/child is sensitized.
- In young patients, food-induced generalized acute urticaria often triggers anaphylaxis. They should be investigated for sensitization to foods suggested by the history, in order to confirm their specific food trigger and, through avoidance of this trigger, prevent subsequent episodes.
- The underlying causes of CSU appear not to be different between children and adults. Thus diagnostic approach should be the same as in adults except possibly in infants.

ANNEXURE

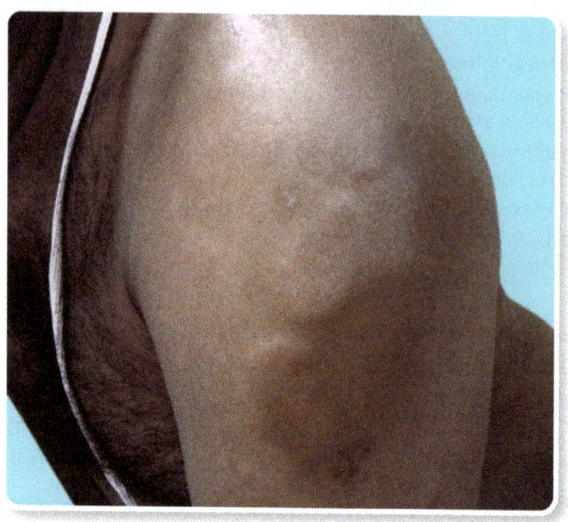

Urticaria Diet

As it is well known that IgE-dependent allergic reaction to food plays a role in acute urticaria specially in children but not useful in chronic urticaria. Only conduction of pseudoallergen low diet can provide information on the presence of chronic urticaria due to food intolerance.

Patient should be informed about:
- Importance of diet
- At least 3 weeks adherence is necessary
- Effect can be seen not until 10–14 days
- Intake of antihistamines and glucocorticoid must be reduced to minimum.

	Foods allowed	Foods forbidden
Basic foods	Additive free bread, potatoes, rice, unprocessed cereals, flour	Cake, biscuit, potato chips
Fats	Butter, plant oils	Margarine, mayonnaise
Milk products	Fresh milk, natural yoghurt, cream without stabilizers	All others
Animal food	Fresh meat	Sea food, seasoned meat, eggs

	Foods allowed	Foods forbidden
Vegetables	Except those for bidden	Peas, mushroom, tomatoes, spinach, olives
Fruits	None	All including dried fruits
Herbs and spices	Salt and onion	All including garlic and herbs
Sweets and beverages	Sugar, honey, coffee, black tea	All sweets including chewing gum, beer, wine, spirits

Prick test:
- This test should be performed in urticaria patients to rule out allergic sensitization.
- In this test about 3 μL of allergen is applied to the skin of forearm and then the skin is pricked with a lancet without breaking the skin.
- Histamine solution and normal saline are used as controls.
- Results are read after 15 minutes. Measure the largest and perpendicular diameter of each wheal.
- To calculate the value largest + perpendicular diameter/2
- Positive reaction means >50% the size of histamine wheal.

Urticaria and Activity Score 7

- An important aspect in classifying urticaria is disease activity.
- Several scoring systems have been proposed but the most widely used scoring system is given below.
- This has to be completed by the patients themselves.

Score	Wheals	Pruritus
0	None	None
1	Mild (<20 wheals/24 hours)	Mild (not troublesome)
2	Moderate (21–50 wheals/24 hours)	Moderate (troublesome but not disturbing daily activities/sleep)
3	Intense (>50 wheals/24 hours or large confluent areas of wheals)	Intense (troublesome with daily activity and sleep disturbance)

[It is recommended that daily disease activity (0–6) is to be documented using the UAS over a period of 7 days, giving a total weekly urticaria activity score (UAS7) of 0–42]

(Limitation of UAS: Not considering the size of urticaria)

Urticaria Control Test

The urticaria control test (UCT) is a validated instrument that can be used by the patients (with either CSU or CINDU) and physicians to assess disease control over the past 4 weeks. Four questions address the control of signs and symptoms of the disease, QoL impairment, efficacy of treatment, and overall disease control. The answer to each question is rated from 0 (very much) to 4 (not at all) and a total score is calculated, where the highest possible score of 16 indicates complete control. A score of ≤11 indicates poor disease control.

CHAPTER
2

Angioedema

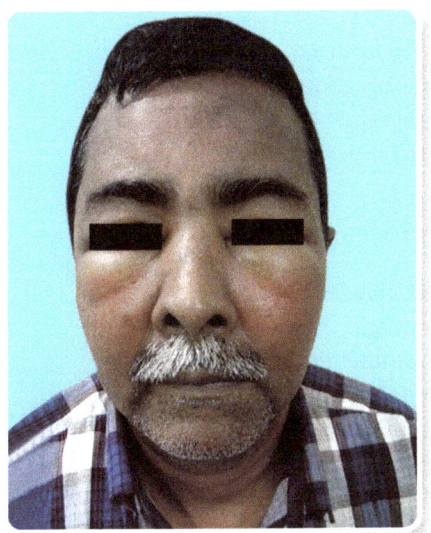

Definition

- It is defined as transient localized swellings of the deep dermis, subcutaneous and submucosal tissues.
- Can be associated with potentially life-threatening episodes of oropharyngeal and laryngeal edema.

Etiopathological Classification

Angioedema without wheals	Angioedema with wheals
Idiopathic (40%)	Similar to urticaria in terms of assessment and management
Allergic	
NSAID induced	
C1 deficiency-hereditary (type 1, 2, 3) - acquired	
Angioedema with eosinophilia: • *Gleich syndrome*: Episodic angioedema with weight gain • Nonepisodic angioedema	
Angioedema due to physical triggers: • Vibratory angioedema • Exercise-induced angioedema	

Pathophysiology

- *Angioedema may be*:
  - Histaminergic
  - Nonhistaminergic
- *Histaminergic type*:
  - Accompanied by wheals
  - Rapid onset
  - Good response to epinephrine, steroids, antihistamines
  - Seen in angioedema associated with chronic urticaria, allergic reactions, cold urticaria, idiopathic angioedema
- *Nonhistaminergic type (bradykinin mediated)*:
  - Lesions progress slowly (subsides within 3–5 days)
  - Poorly responds to epinephrine, steroids, and antihistamines
  - Seen in hereditary angioedema (HAE) and angiotensin-converting enzyme inhibitor (ACEI) induced angioedema.

Hereditary Angioedema (Figs. 2.1 and 2.2)

- Autosomal dominant disorder
- Caused by mutation in C1 inhibitor gene on chromosome 11 **(Flowchart 2.1)**

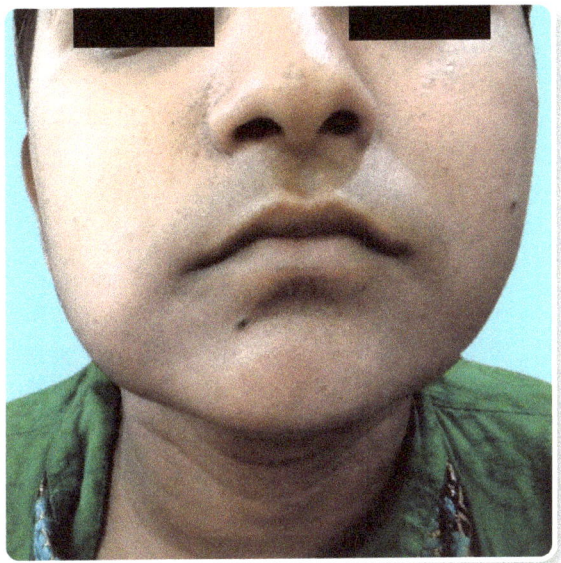

Fig. 2.1: Hereditary angioedema in a young female.

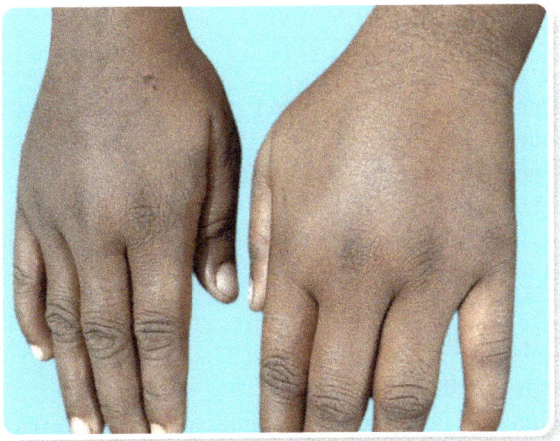

Fig. 2.2: Hereditary angioedema in a lady.

- Prevalence estimated at 1 in 50,000
- C1 inhibitor deficiency leads to bradykinin overproduction which leads to increased vascular permeability and angioedema

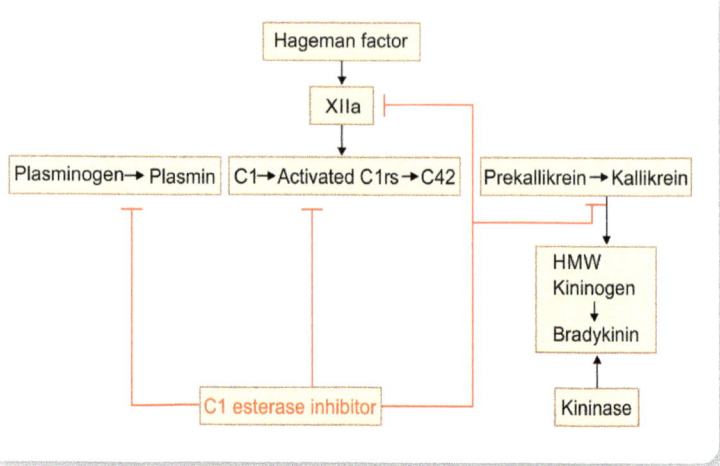

Flowchart 2.1: Mechanism of C1 esterase inhibitor deficiency causing hereditary angioedema.

(By stimulation of Hageman factor generation of plasmin and production of bradykinin occurs. By feedback loop involving C1 esterase inhibitor inhibitory influence takes place over the system. In C1 esterase inhibitor deficiency thus bradykinin is more released leading to angioedema)

- Mainly of two types:
    - *Type 1*: Most common (85%), decreased level of C1 inhibitor about 35–50% of normal
    - *Type 2*: functional inactivity of C1 inhibitor but levels normal or elevated.
    (A third type is called estrogen-dependent angioedema but C1 inhibitor levels are normal.)

Acquired Angioedema
- Very rare condition
- C1 inhibitors deficiency associated with monoclonal gammopathy of undetermined significance (MGUS) and other B cell malignancies
- *Caused due to*:
    - C1 inhibitor consumption by complement activators
    - C1 inhibitor depletion by autoantibodies

Drugs Causing Angioedema
- Two main category of drugs causing angioedema are:
  i. Nonsteroidal anti-inflammatory drugs (NSAIDs) induced angioedema
  ii. ACEI induced angioedema.

NSAID-induced Angioedema (Fig. 2.3)
- Caused by cyclooxygenase (COX) pathway inhibition with overproduction of cysteinyl leukotrienes.
- Usually develops within 24 hours after exposure to the drug.
- Aspirin, diclofenac, indomethacin, and ibuprofen are potent COX 1 inhibitors and have higher propensity to cause angioedema than paracetamol and pyrazolones.
- Indomethacin has the highest propensity for COX1 inhibition and aspirin the least.
- Cross reactivity seen among potent COX1 inhibitors.

ACEI-induced Angioedema (Flowchart 2.2 and Fig. 2.4)
- Offending drugs are enalapril and ramipril.
- Onset usually during 1st month of therapy.
- Late onset presentation seen but usually undiagnosed.
- Cross reactivity with ACE receptor blocker such as losartan seen.

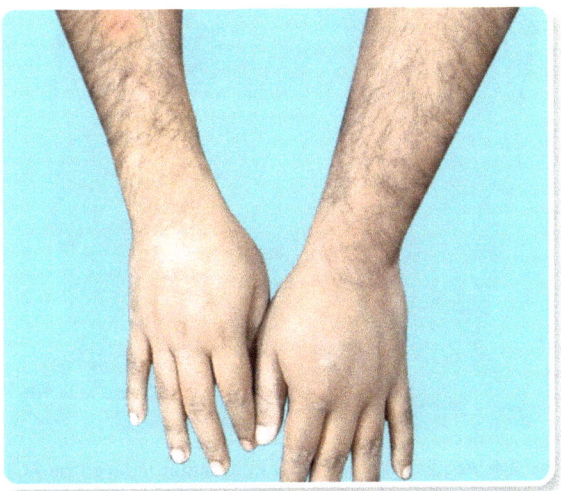

Fig. 2.3: NSAIDs-induced angioedema in a young male.

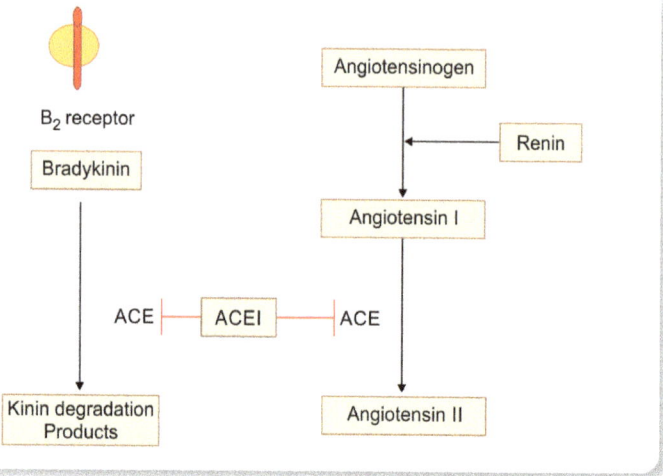

Flowchart 2.2: Mechanism of blocking angiotensin–renin pathway by ACE-inhibitors.

(ACE inhibitors reduce blood pressure as well as breakdown of bradykinin thus leading to angioedema by stimulating B2 receptor on blood vessels)

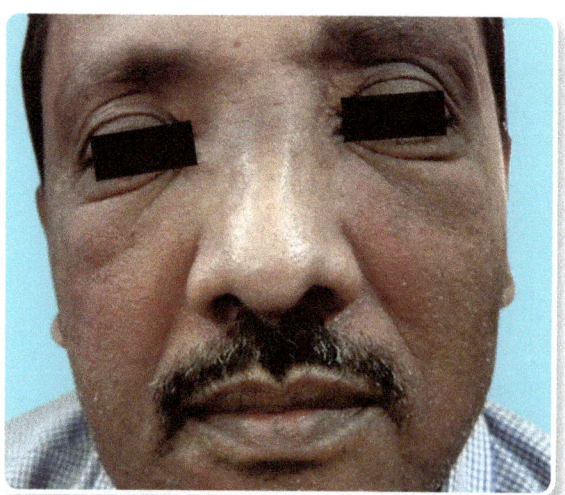

Fig. 2.4: Acquired angioedema in an adult induced by ACE-inhibitor.

Angioedema with Eosinophilia

Two types recognized:
- Episodic
- Nonepisodic

Episodic Angioedema with Eosinophilia

- Also known as Gleich's syndrome
- Characterized by recurrent episodes of angioedema associated with:
  - Weight gain (>18% of total body weight)
  - Fever
  - Marked peripheral eosinophilia (>1,500/mm^3)
  - Elevated IgM
- Carries a favorable prognosis

Nonepisodic Angioedema with Eosinophilia

- Seen predominantly in young women
- Affects mainly bilateral upper or lower extremity

Clinical Features

- Clinical presentation depends on type of tissue affected.
  - *Subcutaneous tissue*:
    - Nonpitting, nonpruritic
    - Affects hand, feet, genitalia and also face with involvement of lips and tongue
    - May be very disfiguring at times
  - *Intestinal*:
    - Presenting with abdominal pain, watery diarrhea
    - Abdominal tenderness present but no sign of peritonitis
    - CT scan shows intestinal angioedema with segmental bowel thickening and ascites.
  - *Laryngeal*:
    - Dyspnea, dysphonia, and dysphagia.
- Characteristic features of few important subtypes:
  - HAE (hereditary angioedema):
    - Manifest usually in children or adolescent
    - Triggered by trauma, stress infection

- Preceded by prodromal symptoms such as headache, paresthesia, flu-like symptoms
- Female patients have more attacks per year and more laryngeal symptoms.
  - ACEI-induced angioedema:
    - Site of predilection includes lower face, tongue, and larynx
    - Triggers include trauma, beesting, and hemodialysis
    - Persons predisposed to develop this subtype include:
      - Afro-Caribbean origin person
      - HAE
      - ACEI associated cough

Differential diagnosis
- Acute contact dermatitis
- Cellulitis
- Melkersson–Rosenthal syndrome
- Cheilitis granulomatosa

Investigations (Flowchart 2.3)

- All patients with recurrent angioedema should undergo screening for C4 level.
- If low then go for qualitative and quantitative assay of C1 inhibitor.

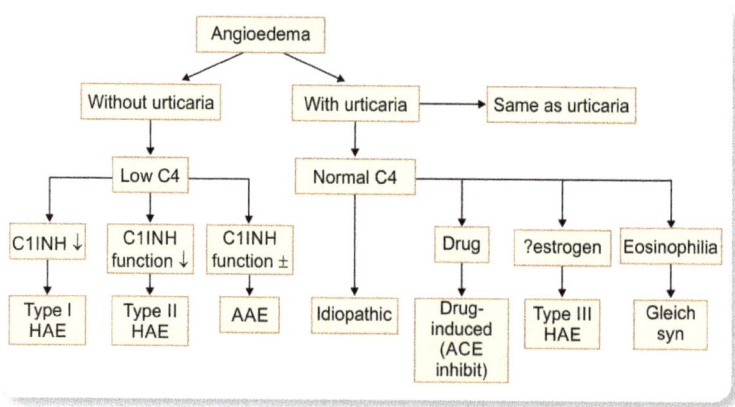

Flowchart 2.3: Approach in a case of angioedema.

(C1 INH: C1 esterase inhibitor; HAE: hereditary angioedema; AAE: acquired angioedema; Gleich syn: Gleich syndrome)

- Elevated eosinophil (>1,500/mm^3) count should point toward Gleich syndrome.
- Screen for underlying B lymphocyte disorders.

Angioedema Activity Score

This instrument can be used to assess angioedema activity, but does not provide a composite score of angioedema, hives, or itch. It includes questions on the occurrence and severity of angioedema as well as its impact on patient's daily activities and appearance. The questionnaire is completed by the patient on a weekly basis, over a 4 week period, and can be used to categorize disease severity as mild (~25 points), moderate (~60 points), or severe (~80 points).

CHAPTER 3

Urticarial Syndromes

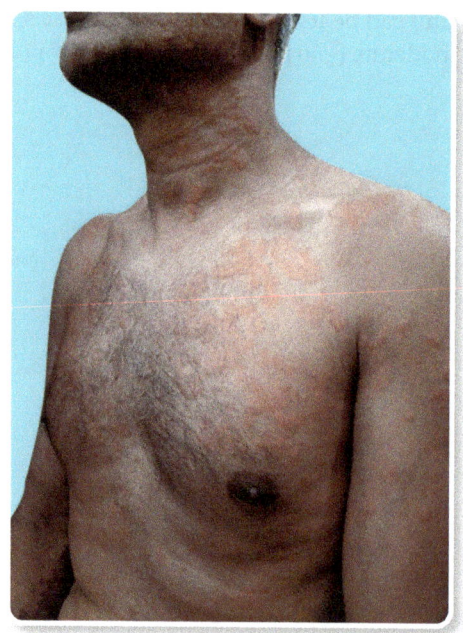

Urticarial syndromes are of two types:
1. Familial
2. Nonfamilial

Familial

- These groups of diseases are associated with urticarial lesions in presence of:
  - Positive family history
  - Neonatal onset
  - Systemic involvement
  - Periodic fever
  - Amyloidosis
  - Neutrophilic predominance in histopathology
  - Lesions are nonpruritic
  - Nonresponsive to conventional treatment

Familial Urticarial Syndromes

Refer **Table 3.1** for detail.

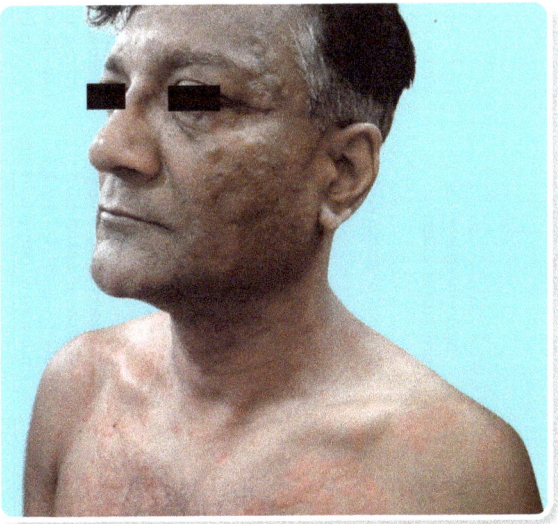

Fig. 3.1: Urticarial syndrome: Familial Mediterranean fever (FMF) in an adult with fever and urticaria.

TABLE 3.1: Familial urticarial syndromes.

Disease	Mode of inheritance	Skin manifestation	Systemic manifestation	Genes responsible	Diagnostic tests
1. Cryopyrin associated Periodic syndrome (CAPS)-3 subtypes	AD			*CIAS1* gene product Cryopyrin	
a. Familial cold induced autoinflammatory syndrome		Cold induced atypical urticarial eruption	Fever, arthralgia. Attacks are almost regular	Same as above	CRP, ESR, genetic testing
b. Muckle–Wells syndrome		Atypical urticarial eruption	Fever, arthralgia. Attacks are almost regular	Same as above	CRP, ESR, serum amyloid A, urinalysis, creatinine level, genetic testing
c. Neonatal onset multisystem inflammatory disease		Atypical urticarial eruption	Fever, arthralgia, sensorineural deafness, renal amyloidosis. Attacks are almost regular	Same as above	CRP, ESR, urinalysis, creatinine level, neurologic evaluation, genetic testing
2. Familial Mediterranean fever (Fig. 3.1)	AR	Erysipelas like erythema at acral sites, atypical urticarial lesions, nonspecific purpuric lesions	Fever, peritonitis, pleuritis, arthritis, renal amyloidosis, meningitis. Variable period between 2 attacks	*MEFV* gene product Pyrin	CRP, ESR, WBC count, serum amyloid A, urinalysis, creatinine level, genetic testing
3. Tumor necrosis factor receptor associated periodic syndrome (TRAPS)	AD	Migratory erythematous papules and plaques overlying areas of myalgia, nonspecific purpuric lesions	Fever, abdominal pain, pleurisy. Average duration of attack 21 days. Number of episodes per year is 6 on an average	*TNFRSF1A* gene product TNF receptor 1	CRP, ESR, serum amyloid A, genetic testing
4. Hyper IgD syndrome (HIDS)	AR	Intermittent morbilliform rash	Arthralgia, abdominal pain, lymphadenopathy. Average duration of attack 1–2 days. Number of episodes per year is 6	*MVK* gene product Mevalonate kinase	CRP, ESR, serum IgD level, urine mevalonate level, genetic testing

(CRP: C-reactive protein; ESR: erythrocyte sedimentation rate; WBC: white blood cell)

Nonfamilial Autoinflammatory Diseases

- This group presents with neutrophilic urticaria of unknown etiology.
- They are usually acquired or polygenic in inheritance.
- Two diseases are described in this category.

Nonfamilial Autoinflammatory Diseases

Disease	Skin manifestation	Systemic manifestation	Diagnostic tests	Treatment
Still's disease	Evanescent erythematous eruption, PG like, rheumatoid nodule like lesions	Seronegative arthritis, hepatosplenomegaly, lymphadenopathy, CNS manifestations, ocular disease	CRP, ESR, RA factor, ANF	Methotrexate, hydroxychloroquine, leflunomide, TNF blockade
Schnitzler's syndrome (Figs. 3.2 and 3.3)	Painful urticaria	Fever, monoclonal IgM gammopathy, bone pain, arthralgia, hepatosplenomegaly, lymphadenopathy	CBC, serum protein electrophoresis	Corticosteroids, cyclosporine A, thalidomide, anakinra

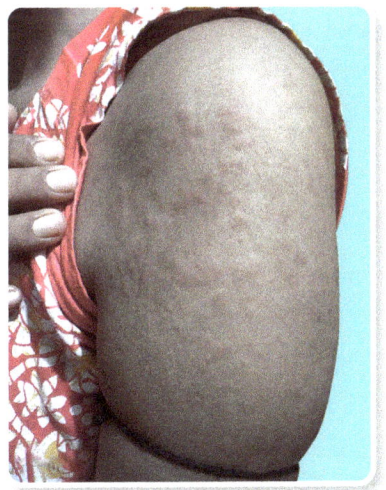

Fig. 3.2: Schnitzler's syndrome: Urticarial lesion in a 21-year-old woman.

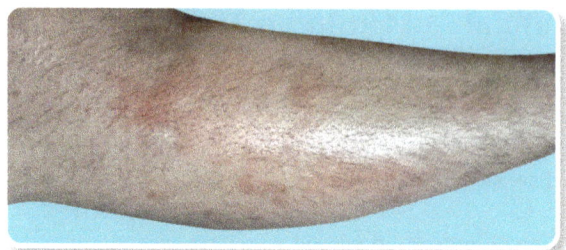

Fig. 3.3 : Schnitzler's syndrome: Maculopapular lesions in a 21-year-old woman.

Other neutrophilic dermatosis with urticaria includes:
1. *Urticarial vasculitis*: Discussed previously
2. Sweet syndrome
3. Behçet's disease

Disease	Skin manifestation	Systemic features	Diagnostic tests	Treatment
Sweet's syndrome	Succulent well demarcated erythematous plaques and bullae	Fever, arthralgia, ocular involvement	CBC, Alkaline phosphatase level, skin biopsy, cancer screening	Systemic corticosteroids
Behcet's disease	Recurrent oral and genital ulcers, uveitis, erythema nodosum	Vasculitis, venous occlusive disease	Slit lamp examination, Pathergy test	Dapsone, colchicines, thalidomide, corticosteroids

CHAPTER 4

Management

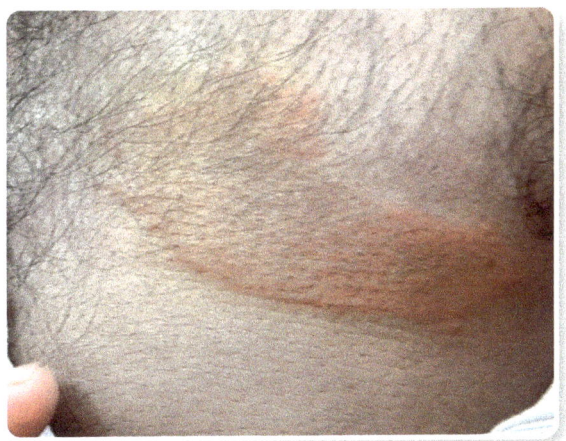

Acute Urticaria

Acute Urticaria: Differentiation from Anaphylaxis
- Acute urticaria and angioedema should be differentiated from anaphylaxis.
- In anaphylaxis, urticaria/angioedema is associated with signs and symptoms in organs other than the skin:
  - The pulmonary tract (wheezing and cough)
  - Gastrointestinal system (vomiting and diarrhea)
  - Nervous system (dizziness and loss of consciousness)
  - Cardiac system (changes in blood pressure or heart rate)

- Epinephrine should be prescribed if the diagnosis of anaphylaxis has not been excluded.

> **Acute urticaria and anaphylaxis**
> Anaphylaxis should always be excluded from acute urticaria. This is of utmost important from prognostic and management point of view.

Treatment of Acute Urticaria

- Antihistamines are effective in most cases and recommended as first-line therapy.
- First-generation antihistamines are rapidly acting but they can produce sedation and impaired motor skills as they can cross the blood–brain barrier. Adult patients and parents of child patients should be made aware of the potential side effect.
- These impairments are less evident or not evident with second-generation antihistamines.
- A brief course of oral corticosteroids may be prescribed in antihistamines refractory patients.

Chronic Urticaria

Monitoring

- In management of chronic urticaria score. The UAS7 to be determined to assess disease activity and response to treatment.

Quality of Life

- To assess the impact of disease on QoL in clinical practice.

Determining the Threshold/Nature of Eliciting Factors

- The threshold of the eliciting factor(s) to be determined to assess severity, for example, critical temperature and stimulation time thresholds for cold provocation in cold urticaria.
- The severity of symptoms and the nature and amount of the stimulus vary from one patient to another. For example, a patient with grass pollen or peanut allergy is asymptomatic when not in contact with the stimulus, and a cold urticaria patient can be asymptomatic in a warm climate. Management should take these variations into consideration.

Basic Approach

- The classification of different subtypes is to be done for proper diagnosis.
- Therapeutic approach is universal and based on the same principles as in other mast cell-dependent diseases in the field of allergy:
    - Elimination/avoidance of the cause or trigger/stimulus
    - Symptomatic pharmacological treatment by reducing mast cell mediator release and/or the effect of these mediators at the target organ
    - Inducing tolerance.

Principles in approach
1. Elimination/avoidance of triggers
2. Symptomatic pharmacological treatment
3. Inducing tolerance

Avoidance of Triggers

1. Drugs
2. Physical stimuli
3. Infectious agents and inflammatory processes

Drugs

- Whenever suspected the culprit drugs should be omitted entirely or substituted by another class of agents.
- Drugs causing nonallergic hypersensitivity reactions (example NSAID) can trigger as well as aggravate pre-existing chronic spontaneous urticaria (CSU).
- Angiotensin converting enzyme (ACE) inhibitors to be stopped in patients of angioedema without wheals.

Physical Stimuli

- Avoidance of physical stimuli for the treatment of physical urticaria is to be attempted but not always practically possible.
- The patient should have adequate knowledge about the physical properties of the respective stimulus to recognize and control exposure in their normal daily life.
- In delayed pressure urticaria/angioedema and in symptomatic dermographism, pressure is defined as force per area.

(Simple measures, such as broadening of the handle of heavy bags for pressure urticaria or reducing friction in case of symptomatic dermographism may be helpful.)

Infectious Agents and Inflammatory Processes

- CSU is often associated with a variety of inflammatory or infectious diseases.
- These infections should be treated appropriately, include those of the gastrointestinal tract, such as *H. pylori*, bacterial infections of the nasopharynx, bowel parasites, intestinal candidiasis, etc.
- In chronic inflammatory processes due to various other diseases like gastritis, reflux esophagitis, or inflammation of the bile duct or gallbladder have been identified as potentially causative for CSU.
- The frequency and relevance of infectious diseases varies between different patient groups and different geographical regions.

Approach in a Case of Urticaria

- Regional differences in causative factors occur in urticaria due to different traditional diets and different prevalence of infections. So it is not necessary to explore all possible causative factors in all patients.
- First step in diagnosis is a thorough history, as described in the Chapter 1 (Diagnosis).
- The second step of the diagnosis is the physical examination of the patient. This should include a diagnostic provocation test including drug, food, and physical tests where it is indicated by history.

Algorithmic Approach

- An algorithm needed (step up or step down) in management of chronic urticaria
- Acute urticaria usually self-limited. Treatment focuses on symptomatic relief
- Complete symptom control in urticaria as safely as possible to be attempted

- For urticaria treatment, as in other allergic or immunologic diseases, an algorithm is needed to both serve the majority of

patients with easy-to-treat symptoms and those being more refractory to treatment.
- The need for treatment within this algorithm may vary over time (step up or step down).
- Acute urticaria differs from all other types as it is self-limited. Treatment is usually focused on symptomatic relief.
- Complete symptom control in urticaria as safely as possible is to be attempted (strong recommendation/clinical consensus following the WHO constitution in conformity with the charter of the United Nations).

Reduction of Functional Autoantibodies

- Little experience in the treatment for CSU by direct reduction of functional autoantibodies by plasmapheresis.
- Plasmapheresis is of temporary benefit in individual, severely affected patients.
- Due to high costs, this therapy is suggested for autoantibody-positive CSU patients who are unresponsive to all other forms of treatment.

Role of Total IgE Estimation and Basophil Histamine Release Assay

- A higher total IgE indicates a higher probability of responsiveness to omalizumab, whereby a normal level indicates higher responsiveness to cyclosporine.
- On the contrary a positive basophil histamine release assay (BHRA) indicates higher cyclosporine responsiveness, while negative BHRA indicates higher omalizumab responsiveness

Dietary Management

- IgE-mediated food allergy rarely cause of CSU
- Pseudoallergic reactions to naturally occurring food ingredients and to food additives seen
- Type I-allergens avoidance clears urticaria usually within 24–48 hours, in pseudoallergy, it may take minimum of 3 weeks.

- IgE-mediated food allergy is rarely the underlying cause of CSU. If identified, the specific food allergens need to be omitted as far as possible.

- In a subgroup of CSU patients, pseudoallergic reactions (non-IgE-mediated hypersensitivity reactions) to naturally occurring food ingredients and in some cases to food additives have been seen. Similar to drugs, pseudoallergens can both elicit and aggravate CSU.
- Avoidance of type I allergens clears urticaria symptoms within 24–48 hours if the relevant allergens are eliminated rapidly, whereas in pseudoallergy, a diet must often be maintained for a minimum of 3 weeks before beneficial effects are observed.
- Success rates may vary considerably due to regional differences in food and dietary habits. More research is necessary on the effect of foodstuffs in causing urticaria, particularly in areas where the daily diet is greatly different from the one in Western Europe.

Role of Specific IgE/Skin Prick Test

Patients with a known sensitization based on specific IgE to food should only avoid these food items if there is relevant information, e.g., double blind oral provocation test or a clear history, to prove that the sensitization has a clinical relevance for urticaria (strong recommendation/high level of evidence).

Role of Pseudoallergen-free Diets

The use of pseudoallergen (nonallergic–hypersensitivity reaction agents) free diets in the extended diagnostic program of chronic spontaneous urticaria has been recommended in patients with daily or almost daily symptoms only (strong recommendation/high-quality evidence).

Inducing Tolerance

Inducing tolerance can be useful in some subtypes of urticaria. Examples are cold urticaria, cholinergic urticaria, and solar urticaria, where even a UV-A therapy has been proven to be effective within 3 days. However, tolerance induction is only lasting for a few days; thus, a consistent daily exposure to the stimulus just at threshold level is required which, for example, in case of cold baths is often not accepted by patients.

Symptomatic Pharmacological Treatment

> **Symptomatic control by antihistamines**
> - The main aim of treatment is the symptomatic relief
> - Continuous treatment with H1-antihistamines is definitely required
> - Some cases may be refractory to H1-antihistamines.

- The main option in therapies aim at symptomatic relief is to reduce the effect of mast cell mediators such as histamine, PAF, and others on the target organs. Many symptoms of urticaria are mediated primarily by the actions of histamine on H1-receptors located on endothelial cells (the wheal) and on sensory nerves (neurogenic flare and pruritus).
- Topical antipruritic agents such as menthol containing emollient can be of symptomatic relief.
- Continuous treatment with H1-antihistamines is of utmost importance in the treatment for urticaria as:
  - Most of symptoms are originated by histamines action
  - Mechanism of action of antihistamines are inverse agonists with preferential affinity for the inactive state of the histamine H1-receptor and stabilize it in this conformation, shifting the equilibrium toward the inactive state
  - Clinical data also support this
  - Safety data are available for use of several years continuously.
- In some cases, especially of CSU, other mast cell mediators (PAF, leukotrienes, cytokines) are also involved and a pronounced cellular infiltrate including basophils, lymphocytes, and eosinophils may be observed. These may respond completely to a brief burst of corticosteroid and may be relatively refractory to antihistamines.

Advantages of Treatment by Second Generation of Antihistamines

> **Modern second-generation H1-antihistamines versus first-generation H1-antihistamines in treatment of urticaria:**
> Modern second-generation H1-antihistamines are to be preferred over first-generation H1-antihistamines in the treatment of urticaria (strong recommendation/high level of evidence).

- The older first-generation antihistamines have prominent anticholinergic effects and sedative actions on the central nervous system (CNS), which last longer than 12 hours, whereas the antipruritic effects last only for 4–6 hours.
- These sedating antihistamines have many interactions with alcohol and drugs affecting the CNS, such as analgesics, hypnotics, sedatives, and mood-elevating drugs.
- First-generation antihistamines can interfere with rapid eye movement sleep and impact on learning and performance.
- The side effects of first-generation H1-antihistamines are most pronounced in promethazine, diphenhydramine, ketotifen, and chlorpheniramine. They penetrate the blood–brain barrier, bind to H1-receptors in the CNS, and interfere with the neurotransmitter effects of histamine. Impairment is particularly prominent during multitasking and performance of complex sensorimotor tasks such as driving.
- Old first-generation H1-antihistamines are a particular concern in the elderly in whom they increase the risk of impaired cognition, inattention, disorganized speech, altered consciousness, and falls. The doses of drugs such as diphenhydramine, hydroxyzine, and doxepin, used in urticaria, are massive compared with the doses actually proven to be effective for the treatment of insomnia (i.e., to produce sedation), for example doxepin 3 mg.
- Modern second-generation antihistamines are minimally or not sedating and free of anticholinergic effect. Drug safety was achieved by the development of the newer modern second-generation antihistamines cetirizine (metabolite of hydroxyzine), loratadine, and fexofenadine, some of which are mostly nonsedating metabolites of earlier sedative antihistamines. More recently, acrivastine, azelastine, bepotastine, bilastine, desloratadine, the active metabolite of loratadine, ebastine, epinastine, levocetirizine, the active enantiomer of cetirizine, mequitazine, mizolastine, olopatadine, and rupatadine have been added to the list of modern second-generation antihistamines.
- Many of these antihistamines have not been appropriately studied in urticaria, and there are considerable clinical differences between them.

- Modern second-generation antihistamines should be considered as the first-line symptomatic treatment for urticaria because of their good safety profile. However, up to date, well-designed clinical trials comparing the efficacy and safety of modern second-generation H1-antihistamines in CSU are largely lacking.

Up-dosing of Antihistamines

Up-dosing of second-generation antihistamines:
A trial of up to fourfold dose of modern second-generation H1-antihistamines as second-line has been recommended in the algorithm of treatment.

- Numerous studies showed the benefit of a higher dosage of antihistamines in individual patients using up to four-fold higher than recommended doses of bilastine, cetirizine, desloratadine, levocetirizine, fexofenadine, rupatadine desloratadine, and levocetirizine.
- Majority of patients with urticaria not responding to single dose will profit from up-dosing of antihistamines.
- Modern second-generation antihistamines at licensed doses are first-line treatment in urticaria, and up-dosing is second-line treatment.

Second-generation H1-antihistamines be taken regularly or as needed?
Modern second-generation oral H1-antihistamines to be taken continuously in the lowest necessary dose rather than on demand (strong recommendation/high-quality evidence).

Different H1-antihistamines be used at the same time?
Preferably up-dosing modern second-generation oral H1-antihistamines that do not cause sedation up to four-fold (strong recommendation/high-quality evidence) instead of combining different H1-antihistamines at the same time (strong recommendation/low-quality evidence) has been advocated.

Algorithmic Approach

Recommended treatment algorithm for urticaria [(The EAACI/gA92) LEN/EDF/WAO guideline 2022].

CHAPTER 4: Management

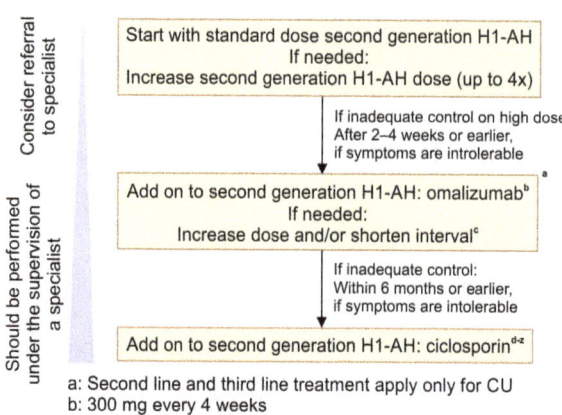

Figure is based on expert consensus and achieved ³70% agreement in the consensus conference

Recommended treatment algorithm for urticaria (Joint Task Force on Practice Parameters by American Academy of Allergy, Asthma and Immunology [AAAAI], American College of Allergy, Asthma and Immunology [ACAAI] and Joint Council of Allergy, Asthma and Immunology 2014)

Recommended step care approach by American guideline
Treatment with hydroxyzine or doxepin can be considered in patients whose symptoms remain poorly controlled with dose advancement of second-generation antihistamines and/or addition of one of more of the following: H2 antihistamines, first generation H1 antihistamines at bedtime, and/or antileukotrienes (step 3).

Step 1:
- Monotherapy with second-generation antihistamines
- Avoidance of triggers (e.g., NSAIDs) and relevant physical factors if physical urticaria/angioedema syndrome is present.
- Begin treatment at step appropriate for patient's level of severity and previous treatment history.
- At each level of step-approach, medication(s) should be assessed for patient tolerance and efficacy.
- Step-down in treatment is appropriate at any step, once consistent control of urticaria/angioedema is achieved.

Step 2:
One or more of the following:
- Dose advancement of second-generation antihistamines used in Step 1:
- Add another second-generation antihistamine.
- Add H2-antagonist.
- Add leukotriene receptor antagonist.
- Add first-generation antihistamine to be taken at bed time.

Step 3:
- Dose advancement of potent antihistamine (e.g., hydroxyzine or doxepin) as tolerated

Step 4:
- Add an alternative agent
- Omalizumab or cyclosporine
- Other anti-inflammatory agents, immunosuppressants, or biologics

British Association of Dermatologists guidelines for the management of people with chronic urticaria 2021 **(Flowchart 4.1)**.

Therapeutic Possibilities for Antihistamines Refractory Patients

- Antihistamines in high dose will control symptoms in the majority of patients with urticaria in general practice.
- Consider switching from one second-generation H1 antihistamine to another in unresponsive patients
- A first-generation antihistamine may be added at night along with second generation at morning.
- Alternative treatments are needed for the remaining unresponsive patients.
- Before changing to an alternative therapy, it is recommended to wait for 1–4 weeks to allow full effectiveness.
- Consider addition of montelukast in addition to second-generation H1 antihistamine in unresponsive patients
- As the severity of urticaria may fluctuate, and as spontaneous remission may occur at any time, it is also recommended to re-evaluate the necessity for continued or alternative drug treatment every 3–6 months.
- Except for omalizumab and cyclosporin A, which both have restrictions due to their high cost, many of the alternative

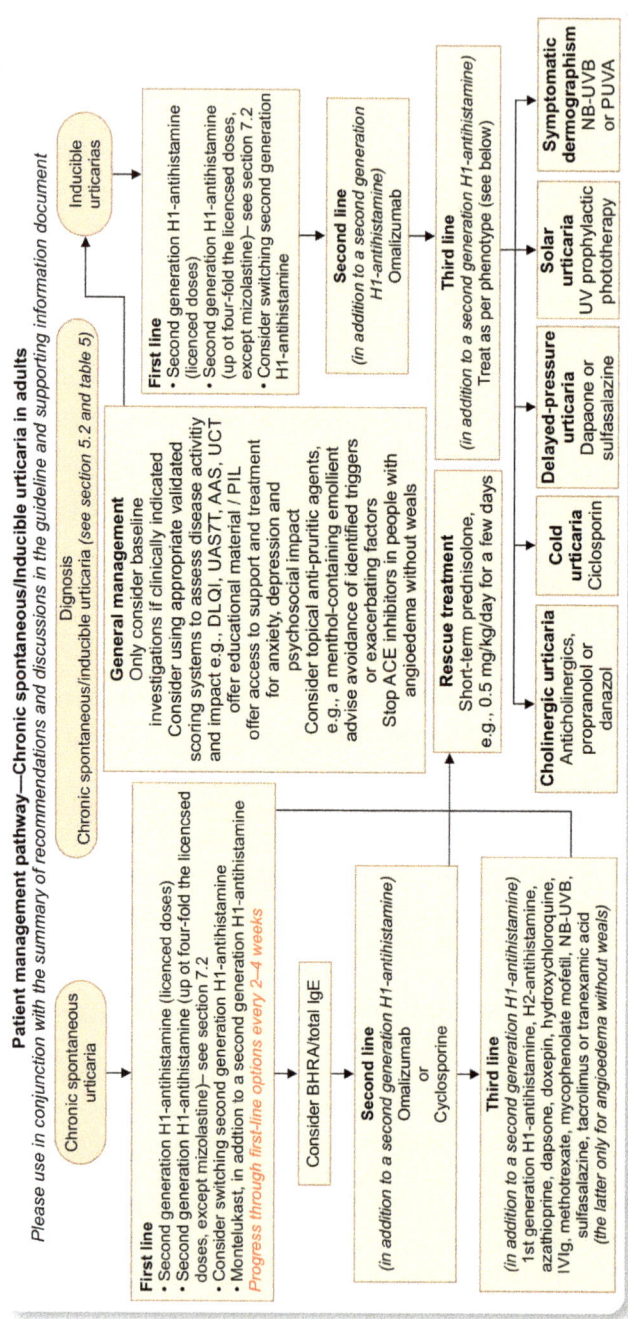

Flowchart 4.1: Patient management pathway for urticaria. For clarity we have divided management options into sections (general treatment, and first-, second-, and third-line options). However, depending on disease severity, disease fluctuation, comorbidities, and national criteria for use of drugs, the order and combinations of treatment may vary and change during each person's disease.

(AAS: angioedema activity score; ACE: angiotensin converting enzyme; BHRA: basophil histamine release assay; DLQI: dermatology life quality index; IVIg: intravenous immunoglobulin; NB-UVB: narrow band ultraviolet B; PIL: patient information leaflet; PUVA: psoralen plus ultraviolet A; UAS7: urticaria activity score summed over 7 days; UCT: urticaria control test)

methods of treatment, such as combinations of modern second-generation H1-antihistamines with antileukotrienes, are based on clinical trials with low levels of evidence. Based on the level of evidence, the recommended third-line treatment options are limited.

- Ligelizumab, a new anti-IgE monoclonal antibody, claims to be more efficacious and needs less frequent administration than omalizumab.
- Dupilumab, monoclonal antibodies targeting the IL-5 pathway, and Bruton's tyrosine kinase inhibitors are all been investigated for CSU.
- Other potential targets include siglec-8 (an inhibitory receptor on mast cell and eosinophil), prostaglandin receptors, and C5a receptors.

Urticaria Refractory to Antihistamines: Algorithm

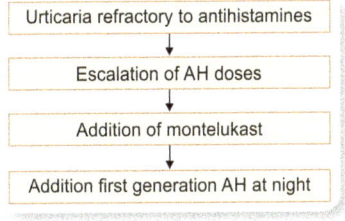

Sources:
1. AAAAI, ACAAI, & Joint Council of Allergy, Asthma, & Immunology 2014
2. Sabroe RA, Lawler F, Grattan CEH, Ardern-Jones MR, Bewley A, Campbell L, et al. Guidelines for the management of people with chronic urticarial. Br J Dermatol. 2022;186:398-413.

Urticaria Totally Refractory to Antihistamines: Algorithm

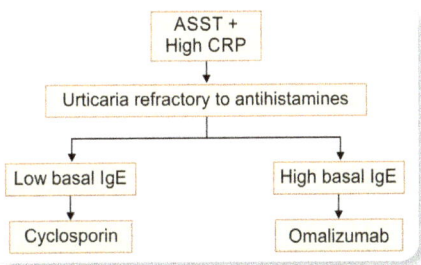

Source: Sánchez-Borges M, Ansotegui IJ, Baiardini I, Bernstein J, Canonica GW, Ebisawa M, et al. The challenges of chronic urticaria part 1: Epidemiology, immunopathogenesis, comorbidities, quality of life, and management. World Allergy Organ J. 2021;14(6):100533.

Omalizumab (Anti-IgE)

> **Omalizumab: Approval in urticaria**
> Omalizumab has been approved in United States in 2014 for treatment of chronic idiopathic urticaria patients who do not respond to approved dose of H1-antihistamines in adults and above 12 years of age. The drug has been conditionally approved in India in same year in same indication.

- Omalizumab has been approved in United States in March 2014 for treatment of chronic idiopathic urticaria patients who do not respond to approved dose of H1-antihistamines in adults and above 12 years of age.
- The drug has been conditionally approved in India in October 2014 in same indication.
- Omalizumab, a recombinant humanized, monoclonal antibody, acts as a neutralizing antibody by binding IgE at the same site on IgE as its high-affinity receptor FcεRI. It reduces IgE serum levels and blocks the IgE attachment to mast cells and other immune cells. Omalizumab denotes a targeted therapy that binds to immunoglobulin E (IgE). It suppresses histamine-induced skin reactions, probably through its reduction of IgE and downstream effects on cellular activation mechanisms. Omalizumab is effective often independently from total serum IgE.
- Dose of omalizumab is 150 mg/300 mg every 4 weekly for 12–24 weeks by subcutaneous injection. Antihistamines or leukotrienes inhibitors may be coprescribed. Side effects are injection site reaction, infection (especially parasitic), thromboembolic events, headache, etc.
- Omalizumab (anti-IgE) has now been shown to be very effective in the treatment for CSU, both in case reports and case series as well as in double-blind placebo-controlled studies in antihistamine refractory selected patients. Omalizumab has also been reported (case reports and small series) to be effective in cholinergic urticaria, cold urticaria, solar urticaria, heat urticaria, symptomatic dermographism, and delayed pressure urticaria.
- Omalizumab should be considered for refractory CU if this is favorable from the standpoint of balancing the potential for benefit with the potential for harm/burden and cost and the decision to proceed is consistent with patients' values and preferences.

> **Use of omalizumab treatment of patients unresponsive to high doses of H1-antihistamines as third-line treatment**
> A trial of omalizumab as add-on therapy to modern second-generation H1-antihistamines as third-line in the algorithm of treatment of urticaria (strong recommendation/high level of evidence) has been suggested.

Cyclosporine

> **Cyclosporine in urticaria**
> Cyclosporin A has been recommended as add-on therapy to modern second-generation H1-antihistamines as third-line in the algorithm of treatment of urticaria (strong recommendation/high level of evidence).

- Cyclosporin A has a moderate, direct effect on mast cell mediator release. It is the only agent of this type to inhibit basophil histamine release.
- It has been shown to be effective in double-blind placebo-controlled studies.
- Efficacy of cyclosporin A in combination with a modern second-generation H1-antihistamine has been shown in placebo-controlled trials as well as open controlled trials.
- This drug cannot be recommended as standard treatment due to a high incidence of adverse effects.
- It is recommended only for patients with severe disease refractory to any dose of antihistamine.
- Cyclosporin A has a far better risk/benefit ratio compared with long-term use of steroids.
- In the context of study limitations, potential harms, and cost, the quality of evidence from the randomized controlled trials supporting cyclosporine is low, leading to a weak recommendation for use of cyclosporine for refractory CU.
- Clinicians need to carefully consider whether administration of cyclosporine is favorable from the standpoint of balancing the potential for benefit with the potential for harm and discuss this openly with patients to determine that the decision to proceed with a trial of cyclosporine is consistent with their values and preferences.

Leukotriene Antagonists

Studies are difficult to compare due to different populations studied, for example, inclusion of only aspirin and food additive intolerant patients or exclusion of ASST-positive patients. In general, the level of evidence for the efficacy of leukotriene receptor antagonists in urticaria is low but best for montelukast.

> **Leukotriene antagonists in urticaria**
> A trial of montelukast as add-on therapy to modern second-generation H1-antihistamines as third-line in the treatment of urticaria (weak recommendation/low level of evidence).

Topical Corticosteroids

In urticaria, topical steroids are not helpful with the possible exception of pressure urticaria on soles as alternative therapy.

> **Topical corticosteroids in urticaria**
> In urticaria, topical steroids are only indicated in pressure urticaria on soles as alternative therapy (low evidence).

Systemic Corticosteroids

- If systemic corticosteroids are used, doses between 20 and 50 mg/day are required with obligatory side effects on long-term use.
- There is a strong recommendation against the long-term use of corticosteroids outside specialist clinics if it can be avoided.
- Depending on the country, it must be noted that steroids are also not licensed for chronic urticaria (e.g., in Germany, prednisolone is only licensed for acute urticaria).
- For acute urticaria and acute exacerbations of CSU, a short course of oral corticosteroids, that is, treatment of a maximum of up to 10 days, may, however, be helpful to reduce disease duration/activity. Nevertheless, well-designed randomized clinical trials are lacking.

> **Oral corticosteroids in urticaria**
> Long-term use of systemic corticosteroids in urticaria has been strongly discouraged (strong recommendation/high level of evidence). A trial of a short course of systemic corticosteroids in urticaria as third-line therapy or as an option for acute exacerbation (weak recommendation/low level of evidence).

Phototherapy

Phototherapy is helpful in treatment-resistant patients with urticaria. For the treatment of CSU and symptomatic dermographism, UV-A,

PUVA, and UV-B (nb-UVB) treatment for 1–3 months can be added to antihistamine treatment.

> **Phototherapy in urticaria**
> Phototherapy can be used in refractory urticaria in addition to antihistamine treatment.

Mycophenolate Mofetil

> **Mycophenolate mofetil in urticaria**
> Mycophenolate mofetil can be well-tolerated second-line therapy for patients with autoimmune and chronic idiopathic urticaria in whom antihistamines and other therapeutic agents have failed.

- Mycophenolate mofetil (MF) has shown benefit in 89% patients of chronic urticaria, specifically 91% of patients with autoimmune urticaria and 88% with chronic idiopathic urticaria.
- Dose of MF ranged from 1,000 to 6,000 mg divided twice daily.
- Mean time to complete control was 14 weeks, ranging from 1 to 31 weeks.
- The drug was well tolerated with no serious infections or laboratory abnormalities gastrointestinal disorders were most common.

Treatment Options in Inducible Urticaria

First line
Same as that for CSU

Second line
Addition of omalizumab in addition to second-generation H1 antihistamine

Third line
Cholinergic urticaria: Consider anticholinergic drugs such as oxybutynin, beta-blockers (e.g., propranolol), or danazol. Even phototherapy may be tried.

Cold urticaria: Consider cyclosporine.

Delayed pressure urticaria: Consider dapsone or sulfasalazine.

Solar urticaria: Advice regarding sun avoidance and sun protection
Consider UV prophylactic phototherapy using the wavelength relevant to the patient, after proper photo investigation.

Symptomatic dermographism: Consider narrowband UVB (a course of 30 sittings usually required)

Also psoralen plus UVA can also be tried

Treatment of Special Populations
Children

- A strong recommendation was made to discourage the use of first-generation antihistamines in infants and children.
- The same first-line treatment and up-dosing (weight adjusted) is recommended as in adults.
- Only medications with proven efficacy and safety in the pediatric population should be used.
- Cetirizine, desloratadine, fexofenadine, levocetirizine, and loratadine have been well studied in children, and their long-term safety has been well established in the pediatric population.
- The choice of the modern second-generation H1-antihistamine in children depends on the age and availabilities.
- Short courses of oral corticosteroids(up to 10 days)can be given in unresponsive cases.
- Omalizumab and cyclosporine approved for in unresponsive CSU in children >12 years but in lower doses than in adults.
- Montelukast better avoided in children as they are more likely than adults to have neuropsychiatric side effects

> **Treatment algorithm in children**
> The same treatment algorithm can be used in children with chronic urticaria (weak recommendation/clinical consensus).

Pregnancy and Lactation

- In pregnancy use of modern second-generation antihistamines is to prefer loratadine with the possible extrapolation to desloratadine and cetirizine with a possible extrapolation to levocetirizine.
- The increased dosage of modern second-generation antihistamines can only be carefully suggested in pregnancy because safety studies have not been carried out and with loratadine, it must be remembered that this drug is metabolized in the liver.
- First-generation agents may be cautiously employed when symptoms demand in the face of nonresponse to modern second-generation antihistamines.

- Use of first generation H1-antihistamines immediately before parturition may cause respiratory depression and other adverse effects in the neonate (the first-generation H1-antihistamines with the best safety track record in pregnancy are chlorpheniramine and diphenhydramine).
- All further steps should be based on individual considerations, with a preference for medications that have a satisfactory risk-to-benefit ratio in pregnant women and neonates with regard to teratogenicity and embryo toxicity.
- All H1-antihistamines are excreted in breast milk in low concentrations.
- Use of second-generation H1-antihistamines is advised, as nursing infants occasionally develop sedation from the old first-generation H1-antihistamines transmitted in breast milk.
- Omalizumab use in pregnancy has shown no evidence of maternal and fetal harm.

> **Treatment algorithm used in pregnant women and during lactation**
> The same treatment algorithm as described in other patients may be used in pregnant women and during lactation in urticaria (weak recommendation/clinical consensus).

Angioedema

1. Management of angioedema with urticaria:
   - Same in the line of urticaria
2. Management of angioedema:
   - Hereditary angioedema (HAE):
     - IV c1 inhibitor concentrate
     - Fresh frozen plasma
     - Icatibant (bradykinin B2 receptor antagonist)
   - Other angioedema:
     - IM epinephrine
   - Acquired angioedema and nonhistaminergic angioedema:
     - Tranexamic acid
   - Prophylaxis:
     - HAE: low dose attenuated androgen

Bibliography

1. Alonso R, Cistero-Bahima A, Enrique E, San Miguel-Moncin MM. Recurrent urticaria as a rare manifestation of familial Mediterranean fever. J Investig Allergol Clin Immunol. 2002;12(1):60-1.
2. Baiardini I, Giardini A, Pasquali M, Dignetti P, Guerra L, Specchia C, et al. Quality of life and patients' satisfaction in chronic urticaria and respiratory allergy. Allergy. 2003;58:621-3.
3. Bernstein JA, Lang DM, Khan DA. The diagnosis and management of acute and chronic urticaria 2014 Update. J Allergy Clin Immunol. 2014:133;1270-7.
4. Bowen T, Cicardi M, Farkas H, Bork K, Kreuz W, Zingale L, et al. Canadian 2003 international consensus algorithm for the diagnosis, therapy, and management of hereditary angioedema. J Allergy Clin Immunol. 2004;114(3):629-37.
5. Byrd JB, Adam A, Brown NJ. Angiotensin-converting enzyme inhibitor associated angioedema. Immunol Allergy Clin North Am. 2006;26(4):725-37.
6. Clemmenson OJ, Menne T, Brandrup F, Thomsen K, Lange Wantzin G. Acute febrile neutrophilic dermatosis-a marker of malignancy? Acta Derm Venerol. 1989;69(1):52-8.
7. Criado PR, Maruta CW, de Avelar Alchorne AO, Ramos AMC, Gontijo B, Santos JBD, et al. Consensus on the diagnostic and therapeutic management of chronic spontaneous urticarial in adults- Brazilian society of Dermatology. An Bras Dermatol.2019;94(2):56-66.
8. Czarnetzki BM. History of urticarial. Int J Dermatol. 1989;28:52-7.
9. Dale HH. On some physiological actions of ergot. J Physiol. 1906;34:163-206.
10. Daschner A, Pascual CY. Anisakis simplex: sensitization and clinical allergy. Curr Opin Allergy Clin Immunol. 2005;5:281-5.
11. Davis AE III. The pathophysiology of hereditary angioedema. Clin Immunol. 2005;114(1):3-9.
12. Davis MD, Brewer JD. Urticarial vasculitis and hypocomplementemic urticarial vasculitis syndrome. Immunol Allergy Clin North Am. 2004;24(2):183-213.
13. Drenth JPH, Boom BW, Toonstra J, Van der Meer JWM. Cutaneous manifestations and histological findings in the hyperimmunoglobulinemia D syndrome. Arch Derm. 1994;130:59-65.

Bibliography

14. Espinosa E, Arostegui KI, Plaza S, Rius J, Cervera R, Yagüe J, et al. Bechet's disease and hereditary periodic fever syndromes: casual association or casual relationship? Clin Exp Rheumatol. 2005;23(38):S64-6.
15. Gimenez-Amau AM, Grattan C, Zuberbier T, Tolubi E. An individualistic diagnostic approach based on guidelines for chronic urticaria. J Eur Acad Dermatol Venereol. 2015;29:3-11.
16. Grattan CE. Aspirin sensitivity and urticaria. Clin Exp Dermatol. 2003;28(2):123-7.
17. Grattan CEH, Francis DM. Autoimmune urticaria. Adv Dermatol. 1999;15: 311-40.
18. Hirschman JV, Lawlor F, English JSC, Louback JB, Winkelmann RK, Greaves MW. Cholinergic urticaria. A clinical and histologic study. Arch Dermatol. 1987;123:462-7.
19. Ishizaka K, Ishizaka T, Hornbrook MM. Physiochemical properties of reaginic antibody: correlation of reaginic antibody with gamma-E-globulin antibody. J Immunol. 1966;97:840-53.
20. Janier M, Bonvalet D, Blanc MF, Lemarchand F, Cavelier B, Ribrioux A, et al. Chronic urticarial and macroglobulinemia (Schnitzler's syndrome): report of two cases. JAAD. 1989;20(2):206-11.
21. Kaplan A, Lebwohl M, Giménez-Arnau AM, Hide M. Chronic spontaneous urticaria: Focus on pathophysiology to unlock treatment advances. Allergy. 2023;78:389-401
22. Kaplan AP, Greaves MW. Angioedema. J AM Acad Dermatol. 2005;53(3):373-88.
23. Kid JM III, Cohen SH, Sosman AJ, Fink JN. Food dependant exercise induced anaphylaxis. J Allergy Clin Immunol. 1983;71:407-11.
24. Konstantinou GN, Asero R, Maurer M, Sabroe RA, Schmid-Grendelmeier P, Grattan CE. The following protocol is recommended by an EACCI/GA2LEN task force. Allergy. 2009;64(9):1256-68.
25. Lawlor EF. The physical urticarias. In: Leung D YM, Greaves MW (Eds). Allergic skin disease. New York: Marcel-Dekker; 2000. pp. 195-211.
26. Lawlor F, Kobza Black A. Delayed pressure urticaria. Immunol Allergy Clin North Am. 2004;24:247-58.
27. Lewis T. The blood vessels of human skin and their responses. London: Shaw; 1927. pp. 21-80.
28. Maurer M, Ortonne JP, Zuberbier T. Chronic Urticaria: an internet survey on health behaviors, symptom patterns and treatment needs in European adult patient. Br J Dermatol. 2009;160:633-41.
29. Novembre E, Cianferoni A, Mori F, Barni S, Calogero C, Bernardini R, et al. Urticaria and urticaria related skin condition/disease in children. Eur Ann Allergy Clin Immunol. 2008;40:5-13.
30. Riley JF. The mast cells. Chapter 16: Mast cells and histamine in the skin. Edinburgh: E & S Livingstone; 1959. pp. 144-59.
31. Roelandts R, Ryckaert S. Solar urticaria: the annoying photodermatosis. Int J Dermatol. 1999;38:411-8.

Bibliography

32. Sabroe RA, Francis DM, Barr R, Black AK, Greaves MW. Anti-FcεRI autoantibodies and basophil histamine releasability in chronic idiopathic urticaria. J Allergy Clin Immunol. 1998;102:651-8.
33. Sabroe RA, Grattan CE, Francis DM, Barr RM, Kobza Black A, Greaves MW. The autologous serum skin test: a screening test for autoantiboldies in chronic idiopathic urticaria. Br J Dermatol. 1999;140:446-52.
34. Sabroe RA, Lawler F, Grattan CEH, Ardern-Jones MR, Bewley A, Campbell L, et al. Guidelines for the management of people with chronic urticarial. Br J Dermatol. 2022;186:398-413.
35. Sabroe RA, Poon E, Orchard GE, Lane D, Francis DM, Barr RM, et al. Cutaneous inflammatory infiltrate in chronic idiopathic urticaria: comparison of patients with and without anti-FcεRI or anti-IgE autoantibodies. J Allergy Clin Immunol. 1999;103:484-93.
36. Salaffi F, Filosa F, Bugatti L, Maestrini MD. Urticaria as a presenting manifestation of adult onset Still's disease. Clin Rheumatol. 2000;19(5):389-91.
37. Sánchez-Borges M, Ansotegui IJ, Baiardini I, Bernstein J, Canonica GW, Ebisawa M, et al. The challenges of chronic urticaria part 1: Epidemiology, immunopathogenesis, comorbidities, quality of life, and management. World Allergy Organ J. 2021;14(6):100533.
38. Shinkai K, McCalmont TH, Leslie KS. Cryopyrin-associated periodic syndromes (CAPS) and autoinflammation. Clin Exp Dermatol. 2008;33(1):1-9.
39. Smith CH, Kepley C, Schwartz LB, Lee TH. Mast cell number and phenotypes in chronic idiopathic urticaria. J Allergy Clin Immunol. 1995;96:360-4.
40. Stojanov S, Kastner DL. Familial autoinflammatory diseases: genetics, pathogenesis and treatment. Curr Opin Rheum. 2005;17:576-99.
41. Toro JR, Aksentijevichl, Hull K, Dean J, Kastner D. Tumor necrosis factor receptor-associated periodic syndrome: a novel syndrome with cutaneous manifestations. Arch Derm. 2000;136:1487-94.
42. Wakelin SH. Contacturticaria. Clin Exp Dermatol. 2001;26:132-6.
43. Wanderer A, Hoffmann HM. The spectrum of acquired and familial cold induced urticaria/urticarial-like syndromes. Immunol Allergy Clin N Am. 2004;24:259-86.
44. Weldon D. Differential diagnosis of angioedema. Immunol Allergy Clin North Am. 2006;26(4):603-13.
45. Yadav S, Upadhyay A, Bajaj AK. Chronic urticaria: An overview. Indian J Dermatol. 2006;51:171-7.
46. Zimmerman AB, Berger EM, Elmariah SB, Soter NA. The use of mycophenolate mofetil for the treatment of autoimmune and chronic idiopathic urticaria: Experience in 19 patients. J Am Acad Dermatol. 2012;66:767-70.
47. Zingale LC, Castelli R, Zanichelli A, Cicardi M. Acquired deficiency of the inhibitor of the first complement component: presentation, diagnosis, course and conventional management. Immunol Allergy Clin North Am. 2006;26(4):669-90.
48. Zuberbier T, Abdul Latif AH, Abuzakouk M, Aquilina S, Asero R, Baker D, et al. EACCI/GA(2)LEN/EDF/WAO guideline: definition, classification and diagnosis of urticaria. Allergy. 2022;77:734-766.

49. Zuberbier T, Aberer W, Asero R, Bindslev-Jensen C, Brzoza Z, Canonica GW, et al. The EAACI/GA2LEN/EDF/WAO Guideline for the definition, classification, diagnosis and management of urticaria: the 2013 revision and update. Allergy. 2014;69(7):868-87.
50. Zuberbier T, Asero R, Bindslev-Jensen C, Walter Canonica G, Church MK, Giménez-Arnau A, et al. EAACI/GA2LEN/EDF/WAO guideline: definition, classification and diagnosis of urticaria. Allergy. 2009;64:1417-26.
51. Zuberbier T, Bindslev-Jensen C, Canonica W, Grattan CE, Greaves MW, Henz BM, et al. EAACI/GA2LEN/EDF/WAO guideline: definition, classification and diagnosis of urticaria. Allergy. 2006;61:316-20.
52. Zuberbier T, Greaves MW, Juhin L, Kobza-Black A, Maurer D, Stingl G, et al. Definition, classification and routine diagnosis of urticaria: a consensus report. J Invest Dermatol Symp Proc. 2001;6:123-7.
53. Zuberbier T, Ifflander JJ, Semmler C, Henz BM. Acute urticaria: clinical aspects and therapeutic responsiveness. Acta Derm Venereol (Stockh). 1996;76:295-7.

Index

Page numbers followed by *f* refer to figure, *fc*' refer to flowchart, and *t* refer to table.

A

Abdominal pain 28
Acquired angioedema 54, 56*f*, 58
Acrivastine 72
Allergic contact urticaria 30
Allergy, type I 16
Ammonium persulfate 32
Amyloidosis 61
Anaphylaxis, diagnosis of 66
Angioedema 1, 4*f*, 5, 35, 51, 52, 58*fc*, 83
   activity score 59, 76
   drugs causing 55
   due to physical triggers 52
   management of 83
   on left side of face 4*f*
   on side of chest 5*f*
   typical 3*f*
   with eosinophilia 52, 57
   with urticarial, management of 83
   with wheals 52
   without wheals 52
Angiotensin converting enzyme 76
Angiotensin-renin pathway, blocking 56*fc*
Anisakis simplex 39
Antihistamines
   cetirizine 72
   first-generation 66, 72
   monotherapy with second-generation 74
   refractory, therapeutic possibilities for 75
   second-generation of 71
   symptomatic control 71
   up-dosing of 73
Anti-inflammatory agents 75
Antinuclear antibody test 45
Anxiety 17
Aquagenic urticaria 29
Aromatic compounds 16
Autoantibody screening 42
Autoimmune connective tissue disease 33
Autoimmune progesterone-induced dermatitis 37
Autoimmune urticaria 17, 18*f*
   diagnosis of 17
Autoimmunity versus autoreactivity 18
Autologous plasma skin test 43
Autologous serum skin test 18, 43, 44*f*
   positive 16
Autosomal dominant disorder 52
Azelastine 72

B

Bacterial infection 15
Basophil 8
   histamine release assay 69, 76
   interact 6
Behçet's disease 64
Benzocaine 32
Bepotastine 72
Bilastine 72
Biogenic amines 16
Blastocystis hominis 15
Blood pressure 56

Blood tests 45
Blood-brain barrier 66
Bradykinin mediated 52
Bruton's tyrosine kinase inhibitors 6, 77
Bullous pemphigoid 38

C

Cells 8
Cellulitis 58
Central nervous system 72
Cetirizine 72
Cheilitis granulomatosa 38, 58
Cholecystitis, chronic 16
Cholinergic
   dermographism 19, 29
   pruritus 29
   urticaria 27, 27f, 81
      disease associations of 28
      triggers of 27
Cold induced cholinergic urticarial 29
Cold stimulation test 25
   negative 23
   positive 23
Cold urticaria 24f, 66, 81
   types of 23, 24
Conjunctivitis 36
Consciousness, loss of 65
Contact dermatitis, acute 58
Contact urticaria 9, 30, 31f, 32f, 46f
   tests for 45
Corticosteroids
   course of 66
   systemic 80
   topical 80
Cutaneous mast cell disorders 38
Cutaneous symptoms 30
Cyclooxygenase pathway, inhibition of 8f
Cyclosporine 75, 79
   efficacy of 79
   in urticaria 79
   responsiveness 69

D

Danazol 81
Delayed dermographism 19
Delayed pressure urticaria 20, 22f, 46f, 81
   detecting instrument 42f
Depression 17
Dermatology life quality index 76
Dermis, superficial 5
Dermographism 9, 20f
   after bath 29
   black 19
   symptomatic 18, 19, 19f
Desloratadine 72
Determining threshold 66
Diarrhea 65
Dizziness 28
Doxepin 72, 75
Dupilumab 6, 77

E

Ebastine 72
Eosinophils 8
Epinastine 72
Epinephrine 66
Episcleritis 36
Episodic angioedema with eosinophilia 57
Ergometric testing 28
Erythema multiforme 37, 38f
Erythrocyte sedimentation rate 41, 62
Exercise-induced anaphylaxis 29, 52
Exertion, physical 16

F

Familial urticarial syndromes 61, 62t
Fexofenadine 72
Flushing 28
Food
   allowed 48
   colorants 15
   for bidden 48

Index

Functional autoantibody 8
  reduction of 69
Functional thyroid disease 16
Fungal 15

G

Gastritis 16
Gastrointestinal system 65
Genes responsible 62
Giardia 39
Giardia lamblia 15
Gleich syndrome 38, 52, 58

H

H1-antihistamines 73
  second-generation 73
Hair dye 31*f*
Hands, swelling of 20
Headache 28, 30
Heat
  and cold urticaria 21
  contact urticaria 9
  urticarial, localized 29
Hereditary angioedema 52, 53*f*, 54*fc*, 58
Histamine liberators, direct 32
Histaminergic 7
Histaminergic type 52
Hydroxyzine 75
  metabolite of 72
Hypereosinophilic syndrome 37
Hypotension 28

I

Illing method, modified 46*f*
Immunoglobulin 76
Immunologic contact urticaria 30, 31
Immunosuppressants 75
Inducible urticaria 41
  chronic 40
  treatment options in 81

Infection 15
Infectious agents 68
Inflammatory bowel disease 33
Inflammatory processes 68
  chronic 16
Insomnia, treatment of 72
Interleukin-3 8
Intestinal candidiasis 15
Intestinal colic 30
Iritis 36
Itchy erythematous plaques 20

J

Jaccoud's arthropathy 35

L

Leukotriene antagonists 79
  in urticaria 80
Leukotriene receptor antagonist 75
Levocetirizine 72
Ligelizumab 77
Loratadine 72, 82

M

Maculopapular lesions 64*f*
Mast cell
  degranulation 26, 29
    stimuli for 8
  liberators, direct 8
Mediterranean fever 61*f*
Melkersson–Rosenthal syndrome 38, 58
Mequitazine 72
Monoclonal antibodies targeting 77
Monoclonal gammopathy 54
Mycophenolate mofetil 81

N

Nervous system 65
Neurogenic flare 71

Neutrophilic predominance in histopathology 61
Nonepisodic angioedema 52, 57
Nonfamilial autoinflammatory diseases 63
Nonhistaminergic 7, 9
 type 52
Nonimmunologic contact urticaria 30, 32
Nonsteroidal anti-inflammatory drugs 8, 55

O

Olopatadine 72
Omalizumab 6, 75, 78
 approval in urticaria 78
 dose of 78
 use of 79
Open application test, repeat 33
Open patch test 45, 46f
Oropharyngeal, life-threatening episodes of 51

P

Papular urticaria 37f, 37
Parasitic infection 15
Pathergy test 64
Periodic fever 61
Peripheral neuropathy 36
Persisting cholinergic erythema 29
Petticoat's pressure 22f
Phenothiazine 32
Photoallergens, suspected 26
Phototherapy 80
 in urticaria 81
Physical stimuli 67
Physical urticarial 16
 tests for 45
 treatment of 67
Plasmin, hageman factor generation of 54
Polymorphic light eruption 26
Polymorphonuclear 8

Polymorphous light eruption 37
Potent antihistamine 75
Pregnancy
 and lactation 82
 polymorphic eruption of 37
Prick test 45, 49
Prophylaxis 83
Propranolol 81
Prostaglandin E2 8
Provocative test 28
Pruritic wheals, development of 24
Pruritus 30, 49, 71
Pseudoallergens 70
 free diets, role of 70
Pseudotumor cerebri 36
Psoralen 76
Pulmonary involvement 35
Pyrazolone 32

Q

Quality of life 11, 40, 66

R

Raynaud's phenomenon 36
Red dermographism 19
Reflux esophagitis 16
Rheumatoid arthritis 33
Rupatadine 72

S

Salicylic acids 16
Schnitzler syndrome 38, 63f, 64f
Sensitize skin 6
Sensory nerves 71
Sjögren's syndrome 33
Skin
 biopsy 36
 manifestation 62-64
 prick test, role of 70
 testing 39
Slit lamp examination 64
Solar urticaria 9, 25, 26f, 81
 associations 26

Spontaneous urticarial 41
   chronic 6, 14f, 17, 67
      diagnostic program of 70
Staphylococcus species 39
Streptococcus species 39
Stress 16, 40
Sweet syndrome 64
Swelling 38
Systemic lupus 33

T

Taste intensifiers 15
Temperature test 25
Thyroid ophthalmopathy 38
Tinnitus 30
Toxocara canis 15
Triggers, avoidance of 67
Tumor necrosis factor-alpha 8

U

Ultraviolet A 76
Urticaria 1, 4f, 81
   activity score 7, 49, 76
   acute 11, 11f, 12f, 65, 66
      diagnosis of 39
      differentiation from
         anaphylaxis 65
      treatment of 66
      triggering factors of 13
      types of 13t
   cells in late phase of 8t
   chronic 11, 14, 66
      diagnosis of 39
      extracutaneous features of 15
      quality of life questionnaire 11
   classification 9
   clinical approach in 11, 42fc
      control test 50
      test 76
      diet 48
      epidemiology 6
      etiopathogenesis 6
      first-generation H1-
         antihistamines in treatment
         of 71
      in children 47
      lesions in presence of 61
      management pathway for 76fc
      oral corticosteroids in 80
      papules 35
      quality of life 11
      recall 37
      refractory to antihistamines 77
      severity of 13
      treatment 68
Urticarial syndrome 60, 61f
Urticarial vasculitis 33, 34f, 35f, 64
   lesions 36
Uveitis 36

V

Valvular heart disease 36
Venous occlusive disease 64
Vertigo 30
Vibratory angioedema 30, 52
Vibratory urticaria 9, 30
Viral infections 15
Vomiting 65

W

Wheal 5, 49
   on elbow, typical 2f
White blood cell 62
White dermographism 19

EU GSPR Authorised Reprsentative
Logos Europe, 9 rue Nicolas Poussin
1700, La Rochelle, France
Phone: +33 (0) 6 67 93 73 78
E-mail: contact@logoseurope.eu

www.ingramcontent.com/pod-product-compliance
Ingram Content Group UK Ltd.
Pitfield, Milton Keynes, MK11 3LW, UK
UKHW021827140426
5217IPUK00016B/1243